The Clinical Nursing Unit

Alan Pearson, MSc, SRN, ONC, RNT, *Diploma in Nursing Education, Diploma in Advanced Nursing Studies. Nursing Officer, Burford Community Hospital and Nursing Development Unit, Burford, Oxfordshire*

Foreword by James P. Smith, BSc(Soc), DER, SRN, RNT, BTA Cert., FRCN, FRSH, *District Nursing Officer, Brent Health Authority, London*

William Heinemann Medical Books
London

First published 1983
by William Heinemann Medical Books Ltd
23 Bedford Square, London WC1B 3HH

ISBN 0–433–24901–3

Typeset by Inforum Ltd, Portsmouth
Printed in Great Britain by Biddles Ltd, Guildford

Contents

Foreword

What will become immediately obvious to readers of this very welcome addition to the nursing literature is that Alan Pearson is unashamedly a nurse — and has tremendous enthusiasm for nursing practice.

In a most commendable way, he has synthesised the thoughts, philosophies, theories and models developed by nursing authors on both sides of the Atlantic to support his own views about the 'clinical nursing unit'.

What is more, he has demonstrated in practice at Burford Community Hospital that nursing knowledge, scholarship and research have relevance for the promotion and delivery of quality nursing care.

The nursing profession needs able practitioners, managers, educators and researchers. Each is interdependent and essential for excellence in nursing, as the author concedes. His book will undoubtedly make a major contribution to the debates and discussions among all nurses about nursing practice developments and the goal of quality nursing care delivery.

The style and content of the well referenced text are enjoyable to read, thought-provoking and exciting.

It is always a particular pleasure to share in the 'launch' of a new nursing author. Even though he points out that the 'purpose of this book is to stimulate discussion on the development of clinical nursing, and not to provide an answer to nursing's most difficult contemporary task', I am sure that Alan Pearson is well on the way to becoming an established author and authority on nursing.

James P. Smith
B.Sc(Soc), DER, SRN, RNT, BTA Cert., FRCN, FRSH,
District Nursing Officer, Brent Health Authority, London

Preface

Contemporary nursing strives to establish a professional orientation to clinical practice both through the intellectual pursuit of nursing knowledge and the institution of practice change. As it does so, the role of the clinical nurse is becoming increasingly analysed and its importance emphasised.

Educators educate for, managers enable, and researchers offer guidance to the practice of clinical nurses. Clinical nurses are those who nurse. Development of the clinical nursing role, and a clinical career structure, is now a subject of much discussion amongst nurses throughout the world. This book is an attempt, through the analysis of nursing literature, to present a framework on which to build a development programme in clinical nursing.

Any book is inevitably the product of every lecture, book, journal, and life event within the experience of the author. So it is with this book, and it seems appropriate to introduce it to you by briefly describing how it came to be.

As part of an academic course, I was required to submit a series of essays on clinical nursing. At about the same time, I was appointed to a new job as nursing leader in a small cottage hospital. This new job was to commence nine months later, and entailed the setting up of a nursing development centre. Having to write the series of essays presented an opportunity to develop my thoughts into some concrete ideas for the new job. Searching the literature and thinking about developing clinical nursing proved to be both exciting and intriguing. Many innovations are occurring, particularly in the USA, and much creativity in nursing can be seen in the literature. In my attempts to outline a development plan, I found ideas with which I could identify, and these ideas formed the basis of the series of essays which was finally written. These essays have become this book; and this book is the working blueprint for the work I am involved in now. As such then, this book represents ideas which are currently being implemented in a real practice situation.

The purpose of the book is to share these ideas to promote more creative thinking and discussion in nursing, and not say 'This is how it should be'. The first chapter reviews the historical growth of nursing so that the current scene is put into perspective. Chapter 2 explores the ideas of advanced clinical roles and suggests a possible structure. A functional unit centred on nursing as a discipline is described in Chapter 3, and the workings of such a unit are considered in Chapters 4, 5 and 6. Evaluating the quality of nursing is discussed in Chapter 7, and Chapter 8 summarises the essence of the book. Whilst the basic proposal underlying everything in the book is the need to establish clinical nursing units, much of what is said is relevant to any ward or department, or any community nursing team. It is hoped that this may be of use to any nurse who wishes to develop practice in his or her own clinical area.

Nursing is a vital human service for today's society, and the strengthening of its practice a duty of all who aspire to providing the quality of care which is the right of all individuals. The proposals in this book may never become a reality, but the beliefs which underly all that is said are rapidly becoming valued attitudes by nurses — a trend which may have a revolutionary effect on those who seek, are directed to, or need the services of nurses.

While in no way wanting to perpetuate the myth that nursing is a specifically feminine activity, and being aware that there is a considerable number of male nurses, the nurse has been referred to throughout the book as 'she' and, in most cases, the patient as 'he'. There seemed no practical alternative to this system, which has been used for ease only.

Dreaming is better than parties

(Tiny Tim, *Beautiful Thoughts*)

Acknowledgements

This book embodies the thoughts, influence and work of many others than me: those patients who have been subject to my attempts to nurse them; my teachers who struggled to badger me out of inactivity; and all those people who have shown me the importance of carrying through an idea without succumbing to the plague of self-doubt.

Special thanks are due to Baroness McFarlane of Llandaff, who supervised me in writing the series of essays on which this book is based; all of the staff of Burford Community Hospital and Nursing Development Unit; William Heinemann Medical Books Ltd; and the following who gave permission to reproduce diagrams in the text:

Nursing Times
Churchill Livingstone
Appleton-Century-Crofts
C.V. Mosby
Little Brown
Collier Macmillan.

My greatest thanks and appreciation must, as always, be reserved for my most faithful and stalwart supporters — Pauline, Andrew and Stephenie — without whom nothing would get done!

1 | The Development of Clinical Nursing: Putting it into Perspective

> To begin at the beginning . . .
> (Dylan Thomas, *Under Milk Wood*)

Before considering how clinical nursing may be developed, it is useful to examine how it has become what it is today, and how the social climate of the time influences nursing.

That group of activities now referred to as 'nursing' probably developed as incidental household duties to satisfy a fundamental need in the family or social grouping — i.e. caring for the sick and weak. In the Western world, nursing has developed as a part of change in society, in the transition from a simple form of social relationships, as in the traditional societies, to a complex form as in today's society. In modern society, relationships are loose and impersonal, as opposed to the importance of emotion and close relationships which was emphasised in traditional society. The community of the nineteenth century was very different to our own present-day translation of the word, and went hand in hand with traditional society. This transition brought about a loss of the previous close ties within the community, and led to anonymity and impersonal relationships, all of which are characteristic of social change. The development of nursing was part of this transition in Western societies:

mother nursing sick in the home
↓
religious caring for the sick
↓
military caring for the sick
↓
professional nurse caring for the sick.

As industrialisation advanced, nursing schools were established to train society's specialists, initially, by the turn of this century, as in the apprenticeship mould. In the USA, some

1

schools were established in the universities as early as 1899, but this is a comparatively recent trend in other parts of the world.

Now, hospitals are becoming more complex, and there is a greater division of labour because of advances in technology. We must consider what we think nurses should be or if nursing should be as it is. Who should nurse? Where? Who should be nursed?

Organising nursing

Beyers and Phillips (1971) say that up to the 1920s and 1930s, the primary effort of nursing was the 'case method' — in which the nurse met the total nursing needs of the patient. The massive expansion of hospital care systems which followed this period brought about a review of the approach to the practice of nursing, and the case method came to be seen as 'expensive in terms of professional nursing salaries, and impractical for most nursing units'. Economic pressures led to the widespread adoption of the 'functional method', whereby tasks were doled out according to ability. The fragmentation of nursing care associated with task assignment eventually became recognised, and the 'team method' approach evolved in some centres, where the care was given by a team of various categories of nurses led by a professional nurse. Currently, there is an emphasis on individualised nursing, with various types of delivery methods to enable this to occur, such as primary nursing (Manthey, 1970, 1973), and the adoption of a systematic, problem-solving approach referred to by many as the nursing process (Yura and Walsh, 1973).

Role of the nurse

Today's nurses struggle to define nursing, and, in so doing, are influenced by a philosophy of nursing which encompasses commonly held beliefs in mankind and health care. Mayers

(1972) suggests that 'Shortly after World War II, when behavioural science theories regarding the "whole person" and "individual differences" became prevalent, nursing accepted the concept of total individualised care as the premise for effective therapeutic intervention. This concept resulted in progress from fragmented disease-orientated nursing care to a more holistic approach for intervention.' Many nurses began to give voice to the view that nurses should move from a medical model of practice to a model conceived for nursing (Roper, 1979; Orem, 1980; Riehl and Roy, 1980; Rogers, 1980). The recognition by many of the need to reform society's beliefs as to the role of women has led to a questioning of the subservience of nurses to doctors and to the criticism of the power of medicine by social theorists (Szasz, 1972; Friedson, 1975; Zola, 1975). Nurses began to assert themselves and seek equality within the health care team. Batchelor (1980) lists a number of factors leading to this demand for equality: the changing status of women; the higher status of nurses as reflected by increased salaries; the enhanced quality of the entry to nurse training; the women's liberation movement; the 'too cosy paternalism' of some doctors; the introduction of a new management structure in nursing in the UK (Salmon Committee, 1966); improvement in the quality of nurse training programmes; the increased number of men in senior positions in nursing; and the rise of trade union involvement by nurses. He sees today's nurses as becoming much more conscious of the specific nature of their professional contribution, and more assertive about their status.

Each nurse plays some part in shaping the history of nursing, contributing to its progression or retrogression. The thinking and actions of nurses are guided by the philosophy of nursing leaders of the time, influenced by other factors – social, medical and scientific. The changes in nursing previously described have occurred as a result of the total situation in a given place at a given time. If contemporary nursing sees its function as far wider than helping the doctor and the traditionally held view of 'nurturing or caring for someone in a motherly fashion' (Weidenbach, 1964), then it does so

3

because of the contemporary thinking in which it functions, and within the context of social change. A consideration of the concept that nursing practice is governed by the needs of the community it serves is of value in understanding the current voiced need by nurses for a radical change in how society perceives the nursing role, and how nurses should perform in such a role.

Effects of community needs on nursing

In its early stages of development, when care of the sick was a charitable undertaking on the part of the nobility, Church and military, and when nursing care was given on a one-to-one basis, expectations were of an affective nature. Nursing was a supporting activity, and medicine was distinctly separate (Friedson, 1975). Those changes emanating from the efforts of Florence Nightingale included gaining status by linking nursing to medicine. Prior to this, nursing was often seen as debasing and possessed little status. Although Miss Nightingale demanded a voice for nurses in decision making in managerial terms, she saw clinical nursing as part of 'what doctor felt was required for the care of the patient' (Friedson, 1975). Scientific and technological advances changed the role of the physician, thus affecting the duties of the nurse, and her role moved from the affective to include various aspects of an instrumental function. By the beginning of this century, nursing had become institutionalised, the nurse was increasingly seen to be working in hospitals, and there was greater control by the physician and formal management by matrons. Community nursing services were separate from nursing in hospital.

Now, the role of the nurse is unclear, and there is much confusion between the affective and instrumental functions, although there is still a retention of the idea of the nurse as a mother substitute and traditional expectations still emphasise the affective role. Davies (1976 and 1977) suggests that society perceives the nurse's role as predominantly affective, with an associated subservience to doctors, and in which

4

accountability for her actions is dissipated. As nursing developed, its attachment to medicine, albeit subservient, lent a degree of dignity, but it is now, according to Friedson (1975), greatly concerned with finding an independent, autonomous role. Although the current drive to implement the nursing process is aimed at improving care standards, its use will enable the identification of unique nursing functions, and accountability for nursing actions is one of its major implications (Kratz, 1977).

Autonomy in nursing practice

In this writer's view, autonomous decision making at the clinical level is notable by its absence. The bureaucratically organised setting of nursing, both in hospitals and in community health, is such that decisions are made according to carefully developed protocols which attempt to cover every eventuality — a feature of bureaucracy (Weber, 1947). This despite the high unpredictability inherent in a service which deals in individuals with infinite possibilities for individual differences. Clinical nurses wish to shed the shackles of bureaucracy, and the management model of practice, and aspire to a professional model allowing independent practice and decision making. Within the last few years, much has been said and written by British nurses about expanding the nurse's role, the development of clinical nursing, and the establishment of an area of autonomy.

Whilst part of the nursing role will always be dependent on the medical diagnosis and prescription, and interdependence within the health team is crucial, autonomy in making nursing decisions in partnership with the patient is seen as an important step towards raising standards. Autonomy refers to the freedom to make decisions within the limits of competence of the individual, rather than having to comply with dictates from superior members of the discipline, or other disciplines. Thus, the argument for autonomy is for 'democratization of the health team' (Christman, 1980), whereby the nurse's contribution is equal to that of the other members of the team.

Advanced clinical role

Ashworth (1975) suggests that there is concern in the UK that standards of nursing are deteriorating, as does the Royal College of Nursing (1979) and many contributors to the nursing press. Since as early as 1932, dissatisfaction has been expressed about the nature of clinical nursing (McFarlane, 1980) and clinical nurses frequently express the need to strengthen the position of those who wish to remain in clinical practice by creating a clinical career structure (Nuttall, 1975; Royal College of Nursing, 1975; McFarlane, 1980). Nuttall (1975) notes that although the terms of reference for the work of the Salmon Committee (1966) did not include the identification of new clinical roles, the creation of the nursing officer was, in part, an attempt to do this; but the nursing staff structure does not, however, place enough emphasis on a need for nurses with clinical responsibility, according to Kerrane (1975b). He suggests that there is a need for nurses within the structure 'to provide leadership in the clinical area whose only commitment is responsibility for patient care', and that this remains an unmet need. Kerrane (1975b) maintains that standards of nursing can only be raised through the introduction of such a nursing role, and the ward sisters are now 'so plaintively' asking 'where do we go from here?'. The Royal College of Nursing (1979) proposes that there is a pressing need for a clinical career structure in nursing because the present structure is 'inappropriate for the clinical nurse because it is bureaucratically and management structured'.

The advocating of advanced clinical roles, and the associated attempt to strengthen clinical nursing, represent a struggle by today's nurses to establish a degree of autonomy in clinical decision making, and opportunities for independent practice where nursing is the central need for the individual seeker of health care, although the interdependent and dependent functions of nurses required for those in need of medical and other care are still accepted. The Report of the Committee on Nursing (1972) states that 'in situations where the curing function (as distinct from the caring function) is subordinate or non-existent, the role of the nurse is central', and it is in these situations that nurses seek the opportunity to work independently. Batchelor (1980) concedes that such situations exist in the areas of geriatrics and psychiatry and suggests that 'nurses would have excellent opportunities to extend their roles in care and to accept an increasing degree of responsibility' in 'forms of care which are alternatives to what has been traditional', which he predicts will emerge in the future as a result of experimentation.

Nursing is on the crusade, alongside other occupations, for professionalisation. Professionalisation simply means the process of becoming a 'profession'. Defining the term profession is problematic, and a wide range of definitions is described by sociologists. Friedson (1975) says that the most strategic distinction of a profession is legitimate, organised autonomy. Occupations which achieve this full autonomy possess high levels of power, and to do this must demonstrate that those involved possess a body of abstract knowledge, and a commitment to service. Seen in this light, professionalisation can be interpreted as a means to achieve power, and the merits of this in relation to nursing are discussed later in this chapter. When society and the other professions recognise an occupation as a profession, professionalism is achieved. Professionalism is thus the state of operating as a professional.

The professionalisation of nursing will only materialise if society affords it such status. Until now, nursing has failed to demonstrate its uniqueness and value to society. Davies (1976) sees the development of autonomy, and thus full professional status, only occurring when the occupation has created a dependency on its service. This 'dependency advantage' has not been part of the occupational strategy of nursing and is not likely to be so if the current 'subordination to doctors, acceptance of a wider range of tasks, and in particular, routinisation' persist. The emergence of an autonomous role in nursing is likely, in its wake, to give rise to major conflict, not least between nurses and the other members of the health team, particularly doctors. The present subservience of nurses is deeply rooted in as much as to give rise to ritualistic behaviour and excessive role portrayal in everyday clinical practice (Stein, 1978). Current day-to-day practice is

7

subject to rule following, standardised activity, and a clear nursing hierarchy with firm allocation of supervisory responsibility (Davies, 1976). Such standardisation is an effective way of avoiding some of the stress and anxiety inherent in the nurse's work, and is partly, suggests Menzies (1960), a social defence system set up by the hospital nursing service 'to protect its members against the stress arising from their work'. Rigid routines are imposed to remove the need for stressful decision making, and nursing schools socialise students into valuing routine. Stein (1978) describes them as being highly disciplined and aimed at inculcating subservience and inhibiting deviance. A fear of independent action results, and the clinging to hierarchical support systems becomes a needed and appreciated activity.

Professionalisation of nursing

If such assertions are accepted as valid, it can be seen that the development of clinical nursing is no easy task, and that the practice of nursing is a product of education and management systems which must be targets for change. The struggle for professional status — the right for active, independent decision making at the clinical level – is likely to be difficult, and be accompanied by interpersonal and interoccupational strife, conflict and anxiety. If it is achieved, nurses must be able to convince society that it is needed, and they must be ready to take the consequences if poor decisions are made by those nurses charged with the added responsibility (Bailey and Clauss, 1975).

The question of whether or not professionalisation of nursing is needed is not easily answered, and it is questionable whether or not some nurses already operate at a professional level. Writing within the North American context, Tiffany (1977) says that although nursing has, for some time now, given increased attention to the education of nurses, to function at the professional level in the clinical situation, and is placing increased importance on clinical nursing, 'nursing has not achieved full professional status and a professional

8

level of clinical nursing does not exist as a norm in the health care system today'. It is postulated that such a judgement can be extrapolated to the reality of British nursing. Some social theorists (e.g. Carr–Saunders and Wilson, 1933) condemn professionalisation as an attempt to attain an elitist position and exert power, and claim that it leads to 'avoidance of accountability to the public, the manipulation of political power to promote monopoly control, and the restriction of services to create scarcities and increase costs'. Full professionalisation leads to the possession of power, according to Tiffany (1977), but although power corrupts, powerlessness also corrupts— 'In the excessive powerfulness of the few, and the patent powerlessness of the many, oppression flourishes'. If the professionalisation of nursing is a bid for power, it is necessary to view this bearing in mind the truism that power itself is not inherently evil. A shift in the balance of power within the health care system of today, to allow for the increasing possibility of nurses making decisions about the nursing needed by an individual, is a move which may very well have a beneficial effect in health care. Allowing the nurse the freedom for autonomous decision making in nursing situations at the clinical level is about professionalisation— and this, in turn, is about the power to act independently when those functions which are uniquely nursing are demanded by the patient's needs.

The professionalisation of nursing may lead to the pluralisation of elite health care occupations, and the resulting equalisation of power amongst those occupations is likely to increase the number of viable options available to those who seek health care (Tiffany, 1977). Ashley (1975) comments that, in nursing, 'second class citizenship has brought about second class professionalism'. To deliver the nursing deserved by mankind, nurses may need to attain 'first class citizenship' in order to give 'first class nursing' through equalising the power distribution which exists at present. Bhola (1975) purports that 'to *be* is to be able to experience power . . . to *be* is to be *powerful*'.

Contemporary nursing strives to affirm its unique contribution to health care; to proclaim its right for an area of independent practice; to appeal for a move towards the development of clinical nursing and expansion of the nursing role. This book attempts to describe *creatively* a framework for the development of clinical nursing based on theoretical concepts drawn from nursing literature, and then applied to the reality of current clinical practice. As such, it hopes to serve as a basis for discussion to stimulate the realisation of the aspirations of those nurses who earnestly seek to deliver a standard of nursing which they believe is the right of all individuals, through the establishment of advanced, expanded, professional clinical roles in nursing, and thus enhanced status to those who choose to pursue a career with direct patient involvement.

2

Developing New Clinical Roles in Nursing: the Consultant in Clinical Nursing

> Since the nursing profession is striving to develop a unified holistic theory for practice, a commitment to provide a unified role for nursing (which encompasses service, education, research and consultation) should be compatible.
>
> (S. Spiloto, *A Unified Role for Nursing*)

No matter how much experience, training, or education a nurse acquires, status and higher financial rewards can only be hers if she chooses to desert the practical reality of clinical nursing and join the ranks of nursing's elite— the managers and educators. The 'key' nursing role is that of the sister/charge nurse (Pembrey, 1980), yet it remains the lowest grade of registered nurse with the exception of the staff nurse. Nuttall (1975) maintains that 'the advanced knowledge and skills possessed by some nurses receive no formal recognition as there are no established clinical posts which identify the exceptional contribution which such nurses are able to make, and encourage the enlargement of that contribution.' McFarlane (1980) concurs with this, and says that 'there should be career opportunities in clinical nursing comparable to those in nurse teaching and management.' This implies that clinical nurses should have the opportunity to occupy positions on a par with those presently held at the highest level, without deserting the clinical arena where nurses and patients interact to overcome nursing problems.

How can such a suggestion materialise, and how is such a proposal being approached? Much discussion has taken, is taking, and will be taking place on developing a career structure for clinical nursing. In the USA, new initiatives are already being implemented, but in the UK, concrete proposals have yet to be seen by the clinical nurses who are seeking recognition of their central role. The same situation exists in many other countries where a hierarchical structure exists in nursing. Published literature on the subject of a career ladder for clinical nurses is ambiguous and confusion reigns over what is meant by the role titles created for existing and advanced clinical roles, with no clear, generally acceptable thinking being generated for nursing's consideration. The greatest ambiguity lies in the interpretation of the terms 'expanded' and 'extended' roles, and 'clinical nurse specialist' and 'clinical nurse consultant'.

Extension and expansion

Zornow (1977) sees extension as 'elongating specific, already assumed functions to fill perceived gaps', and MacGuire (1980) suggests that it refers to the situation where nursing expertise is not vital and the additional tasks incorporated in the widening of the role are essentially medical. Expansion is a fundamentally different concept, and is more concerned with a 'deepening' and development of the role, drawing on those skills and areas of knowledge which are uniquely nursing.

Extended roles are not new, and there is now a rapid acceleration in creating new extended roles in nursing. They widen the nurse's role to include various tasks which were previously seen to be the domain of doctors. McFarlane (1980) suggests that such innovations require the nurse to acquire basic diagnostic skills for which she 'is not at present trained (but for which she could be trained)'. The occupier of extended roles therefore practises on the basis of a medical model of care (McFarlane 1980):

diagnosis ——————————⟶ treatment ——————————⟶ cure
(of disease)

Many such roles have been described, particularly from within the North American context. The nurse practitioner is a nurse who receives preparation to take health histories, carry out physical examinations, work in a colleague relationship with doctors, and to carry out dependent and independent functions. This type of nurse is now increasingly becoming part of American health care systems, operating in defined areas such as paediatrics, geriatrics, psychiatry, and primary health care (MacGuire, 1980). Nurse practitioners are known as paediatric nurse practitioner, geriatric nurse practitioner, psychiatric nurse practitioner, and family nurse practitioner. The primex nurse fulfils a similar function, acting as a primary nurse practitioner who makes health assessments, and independently assumes responsibility and accountability for prevention of, and dealing with, common health problems of patients. In addition, nurses are assuming roles which do not necessarily require previous nursing knowledge or expertise, such as those of 'health associate, practitioner associate, associate physicians, physician assistant, Medex' and others (MacGuire, 1980). It is apparent that the development of these types of roles stems from an attempt to alleviate the shortage of medical manpower in certain fields, rather than from a desire to develop nursing itself. MacGuire (1980) sees a similar pattern beginning in the UK, citing the example of district nurse attachment to the community health practices described by Marsh. The role of the district nurse in the practice described appears to be the same as that of the nurse practitioner, and its development seems to have had a desirable effect on health care delivery. Extending the nurse's role in this way may well be a vital need in today's community, and, if this is so, may be a move with which nurses must be prepared to experiment. However, extension in this way is often met with concern and disapproval by nurses. MacGuire (1980) describes two prevalent schools of thought on extending/expanding the nurse's role. In the first, 'Model A', nursing and medicine are seen as entirely separate, nursing aiming at 'care' and medicine at 'cure'. Supporters of this model express the fear that the essential, fundamental nursing functions will be lost in the new emphasis on the nurse performing medical tasks. 'Model B' is based on the assumptions that health care can be delivered by any health care worker regardless of discipline, as long as they are appropriately trained, and that nurses who are specially trained are 'as good as or at least not worse than, the doctor'. If 'Model B' is accepted, then the role of nurse practitioner and other similar roles are to be favoured and encouraged. If, however, 'Model A' is the one of choice, the extended role is opposed, and the call is for expansion of the nursing role.

It can be argued that both models can be supported. It may be appropriate to extend nurses' roles in some clinical contexts to ensure an adequate distribution of services, whilst expanding roles in other contexts to improve nursing, in its purest sense, by building up nursing knowledge and equipping nurses to provide nursing expertise for those who need it. Such a view is acceptable if the purpose of nursing is to meet the needs of the contemporary society which it serves. The danger is, however, that extending the nursing role may be emphasised and encouraged at the expense of expanding it.

Hall (1964) says that the medical aspect of nursing has grown and grown so that something had to go: 'What went was the nurturing process which now the nurse in turn delegated to less well prepared persons.' She observes that nurses have shed the essentially 'nuturing' aspects of their role to practical nurses, but that doctors have not yet established a cadre of practical doctors. 'They don't need them . . . they have nurses. Interesting too, is the fact that most nurses show by their delegation of nurturing to others, that they prefer being second class doctors to being first class nurses. If she feels better in this role, why not? This is the perogative of any nurse. One good reason why not for more and more nurses is that with this increasing trend, patients receive from professional nursing, second class doctoring; and from practical nurses, second class nursing. Some nurses would like the public to get first class nursing.'

A difficult dilemma stares us in the face. To extend, and not expand, the nurse's role, because that is what the seekers of health care need? To expand, and not extend, because they need that even more? Or is it possible to do both? Extended roles are needed, and if nurses do not respond to the need, others are willing to step in and increase the ever-growing army of technicians which proliferate in the health care system to confuse the patient with highly fragmented care. Some extended nursing roles must be maintained, and created.

14

For the service of nursing itself, however, expansion of its uniqueness is crucial for its development and future existence. Expansion is the major challenge for nurses themselves, and the creation of a clinical career structure must be based on this aspect of the role change.

McFarlane (1980) asserts that 'the caring role of the nurse has been so neglected that this needs expansion (in depth)', and that the nursing model of care needs to be more adequately developed:

assessment ⟶ help ⟶ self-care
(of self-care disabilities)   (assistance, etc.)

The primary aim of this book is to explore the expansion of the role of the nurse and to offer a framework on which to base a clinical career structure in nursing, accommodating expanded roles.

The unique role of the nurse transcends boundaries of medical specialities, age groups, and health care settings — there is a common element in all forms of nursing, and it is this care which is exclusive to the nurse above all others. None of the British literature reviewed describes the development of an expanded, independent role based on the 'speciality' which seems so 'unspecial' — the unique nurturing, comforting, caring, encouraging and facilitating part of nursing which is its very essence. There is thus an apparent need for earnest and creative attempts to re-establish the central importance of this aspect of nursing, and proclaim nursing's primacy at it.

Nurse specialists and consultants

In discussing proposed expanded roles in nursing, the terms 'clinical nurse specialist' and 'clinical nurse consultant' are most frequently used (Royal College of Nursing 1971, 1975, 1979). There is obvious confusion about what these terms mean, and what, if any, the differences are between them.

The clinical nurse specialist is succinctly defined as 'an

expert practitioner of nursing with considerable knowledge and a high degree of skills and extensive experience in the care of patients in the speciality concerned. She would introduce new nursing practice by improving nursing techniques and working out better ways of performing current nursing care.' Such roles are appearing in the National Health Service in Britain today, and are seen to be playing an important part in the improvement of care delivery (Burdge, 1978; Cox, 1978). The crucial word in the role title is specialist— the implication being that the nurse occupying the role has experience in a special area— a piece of the whole which comprises total care. A variety of specialists has been developed, based on medical diagnosis, procedures, and specific aspects of nursing care, e.g. groups and settings for care. Examples are clinical nurse specialists in: paediatrics, oncology, stoma care, intravenous therapy, nutrition, and many others. In effect, the nurse develops expertise in a defined field, and offers guidance to the givers of total care, whilst also solving problems within the defined field by direct action. No set minimum standards of professional preparation are laid down for specialist roles, although the Royal College of Nursing (1975) suggests a post-basic qualification and the Diploma in Nursing of the University of London as desirable requisites. It is conceivable that a clinical nurse specialist may be either a pure specialist with responsibilities only for the special area, or a general nursing care giver who has developed specialist expertise and is available for consultation by others, and who can be assigned to give total care to a patient who has a need for her expertise. There are endless opportunities to develop specialities within nursing, and the idea of encouraging specialisation is open to argument. Perhaps the principle of assigning nurses to give comprehensive nursing to a patient, at present gaining increasing support from nurses, demands a support team of nurse specialists to advise and assist those nurses whose task it is to give total care.

The term clinical nurse consultant is used by many and it is difficult to identify the difference between this role and that of the clinical nurse specialist. Indeed, Ashworth (1975) argues that the name is unimportant, and does not differentiate between the two. It is postulated that there is a need for a further expanded role in addition to the clinical nurse specialist, and that this is the clinical nurse consultant. Kohnke (1978) identifies a role for nurses who have a wider educational preparation than that previously suggested for the clinical nurse specialist. It is the role of a consultant, in its truest sense, and a need for such a role is apparent in Britain. The role described by Kohnke is independent and is that of an expert resource consultant undertaking consultation in its pure form, i.e. offering advice and accepting patients for care when required. The nurse is a consultant in the process of nursing; an expert in meeting the nursing needs of individuals who will accept patients and participate in this process when asked to do so, whilst advising others on their work on request. As such, the consultant specialises only in nursing, and its independent practice for patients whose sole need is nursing. As nursing progresses, it may identify its major specialities, for example child nursing, adult nursing, nursing the elderly, but it is proposed that the present need is for a nurse in each health district or division who is able to be consulted and asked to care for patients with nursing problems. Thus, the major distinction between the specialist and consultant is that the former works in a collaborative role, and the consultant works independently. The specialist will most frequently be concerned with the care of patients who are primarily seen to be under medical treatment or surveillance. Kohnke (1978) suggests that the consultant be prepared to masters degree level, and a high degree of expertise and knowledge is vital if the consultant is to establish what Sheahan (1972) sees as the main role of the consultant — establishing 'a new nurse–patient relationship comparable in quality and distinction to that which presently exists between the physician and his patient'. For a real consultant role, access to beds is needed, except in the area of community nursing, and complete autonomy in clinical decision making granted. Such a move is likely to arouse hostility and suspicion, not least from doctors. Kerrane (1975b) argues a need for change in medical attitudes to nursing by re-education to allow the development of advanced nursing roles. His assessment of doctors' current

17

attitudes towards nurses concludes with 'the ignominity of the position would not be tolerated by the American nurse specialist who justly insists on a "colleague relationship" with the doctor at all times.'

That extended roles for nurses are to be encouraged is not denied, but the emphasis here is that expansion of the nursing role to enable greater independence in the practice of nursing and a career structure for clinical nurses is of increasing importance to patient care. The theoretical and conceptual discussion may now be applied to describe a framework for such a structure.

Clinical career structures

The major difficulty in introducing new clinical roles lies in integrating them into the existing structure. This difficulty is compounded by the current uncertainty regarding how best to organise a management structure in nursing. It is therefore essential to view the following discussion bearing in mind that present structures are likely to change; a huge variety of structures exists throughout the world; a great deal of evaluative research on structuring management in nursing is warranted; and there is wide variation in how nurses envisage re-organisation of authority.

As far as re-organisation is concerned, there is now an emphasis on basing the organisation of health care on small units, and Gonzalez (1981) outlines a new structure at this unit level, applicable to British nursing, but transferable to nursing anywhere within an organisational setting. He sees a need to abandon intermediate management levels. In their place he suggests a unit head, referred to as the director of nursing services, leading a team of senior and junior sisters, or head nurses, with line authority. In addition, he suggests that a number of nurses in 'staff' positions should be appointed, being directly responsible to the director, and being delegated the task of advising the director, senior sisters, and junior sisters. Gonzalez's (1981) structure is presented in Fig. 1. The concepts of line authority and staff authority are highly

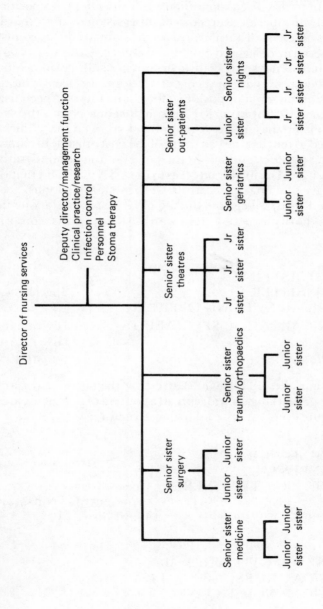

Fig. 1 Unit organisation chart (after Gonzalez, 1981).

relevant to this discussion. Line authority refers to a position whereby a superior exerts direct supervision over a subordinate, whereas staff authority gives the right to advise, counsel and perform delegated functional duties. Gonzalez (1981) sees clinical nurse specialists occupying staff positions, but makes no provision for a consultant level. In discussing the merits of line or staff positions for clinical nurse specialists, Kerrane (1975b) says 'My personal feeling is that the staff relationship has more to commend it ... One clinician stressed to me that the "strength of the post must be in clinical nursing practice and not in the power of the administrative authority".' During a study trip to the USA, he found that the majority of clinical specialists were in staff positions.

The Royal College of Nursing (1979) proposes a four-tier line authority structure from ward sister upwards, comprising:

WARD SISTER II
WARD SISTER I   } Specialists
CLINICAL NURSING OFFICER
CLINICAL NURSE SPECIALISTS   Divisional
                              District Area
                              (as required)

McFarlane (1980), whilst stressing the need for research before embarking on widespread adoption of a clinical career structure, suggests the following structure:

NURSING AIDE
TRAINEES
NURSE PRACTITIONER (a) Generalists — equivalent
                      to present Staff Nurse and
                      Ward Sister II

NURSE PRACTITIONER (b)
CLINICAL NURSE SPECIALIST
CLINICAL NURSE CONSULTANT

She describes the first four grades as those which form the ward clinical nursing teams. The clinical nurse specialist is described as a 'specialist equivalent in grading to a ward sister I or nursing officer'. The clinical nurse consultant may be appointed at levels 'depending on content and span of consultancy work. The salary would be negotiable on the basis of job content and evaluation up to the area level and the lines of responsibility would be dictated by the level of appointment. For example, the role of area nurse (child health) would readily be developed into a consultancy role over the whole field of child health in hospital and community.'

It is difficult to decide whether the two advanced clinical roles suggested here, of clinical nurse specialist and consultant in clinical nursing, should have line or staff relationships. Kerrane (1975b) reports that there is strong feeling amongst American nurse specialists themselves that they must work in staff posts. They feel that they must be without line responsibilities if they are to fulfil their roles. However, the prevailing hierarchical structure in nursing may demand that any newly created clinical roles must fit into a 'slot' provided by the structure. Specialists and consultant roles are derived from a perspective of nursing focusing on a professional model of practice, whereas a management model approach is the one largely embraced at the moment. Kramer (1974) and Kohnke (1975) point out how hospitals are at present not structured to absorb a professional model of practice. If increased education and experience are demanded for specialists, and academic qualifications for consultants, then it is essential that the salaries for the post must reflect this. With the existing salary system related to a hierarchical structure, it is perhaps necessary to equate advanced clinical roles with managers and teachers. The nurse specialist needs to be equated with middle-level managers and teachers, and the consultant with high-level managers and teachers. It would appear, at this stage in the development of nursing, that the implementation of a pilot scheme utilising the proposals of McFarlane (1980b) or the Royal College of Nursing (1979) is a necessary prelude to the provision of a system of career progression for clinical nurses. In addition, the relationship between the

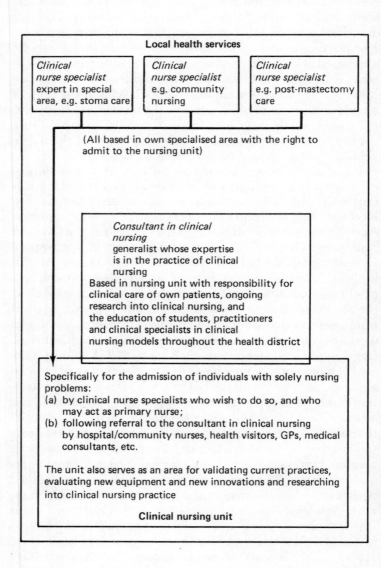

Fig. 2 Relationship between the clinical nursing unit and the local health services.

proposed consultant in clinical nursing, clinical nurse specialist, and the clinical nursing unit needs consideration. It is proposed that the clinical specialist should relate closely to the clinical nursing unit, and that it should be possible for her to be able to admit her own patients to the unit for further care under her supervision when medical needs preclude the necessity of admission to the ward. Figure 2 attempts to clarify how the CNU may relate to the wider health district, and the clinical nurse specialists in areas such as community nursing, oncology, stoma care etc.

Colloquially, there is a growing opinion that the creation of clinical grades above the level of ward sister/charge nurse will serve to devalue the role. Sisters themselves suggest that they are the clinical experts. They propose that the sister grade should remain as the highest clinical grade, but that increased financial rewards should be given based on the merit-award system currently in use for medical consultants. Little documentation on this system exists, but perhaps merit awards could be given on the basis of such things as research activity, publications, and the possession of academic awards. Although these mooted suggestions merit some consideration, major problems are evident. The ward sister's role has been shown by many empirical studies (e.g. Pembrey, 1980) to be extremely complex, and the possibility of a ward sister being available for consultation, either as a specialist or clinical consultant, seems to be unlikely because of her mammoth task in 'running' her ward or department, and the same seems to be true in the case of the district nursing sister.

It is therefore postulated here that four levels of clinical nurses are required to provide effective nursing to those who seek it, based on the proposals of the Royal College of Nursing (1979) and McFarlane (1980b), and that these levels should be equated with the career structure for teachers and managers.

The largest group of nurses is that of the direct care givers in situations where a largely collaborative function is required. This may be a hospital ward for surgical patients, or a community nursing unit, for example. The level-one nurses may be equated with the existing staff nurse grade, and the level two with the ward sister/charge nurse/community nursing sister etc.

The third level is that of the clinical nurse specialist, who has gained expertise in a specialised area such as terminal care, community paediatric care etc. This level can be equated with teaching and intermediate management grades.

The fourth is the consultant in clinical nursing, who is appointed to a large hospital, a local health service grouping etc. and can be equated to those nurses at present occupying posts at top management education levels. It is this new role, as yet not realised in Britain, which is seen to be crucial to the development of clinical nursing, and the 'top of the ladder' for clinical nurses. The consultant in clinical nursing will be a true practitioner who nurses in reality, acts as a teacher to nurses, a consultant for nurses, a representative of clinical nurses at the top management level, and an initiator, interpreter and encourager of clinical nursing research. It is a concept with endless possibilities, and an exciting challenge to be grasped by those who wish to develop clinical nursing. McFarlane (1980b) describes the nurse consultant as a 'specialist whose expertise and knowledge qualifies her to be consulted by other nurses and who gives advice on standards of care. The knowledge base, research and teaching functions are more highly developed.' She adds that some posts could be occupied by educators, as in joint appointment schemes which are emerging, and stresses that the present basic training is not adequate for this level of worker, and that appointing those without extra preparation would 'bring the scheme into disrepute'.

It is accepted that major difficulties will undoubtedly arise in the integration of these two higher level clinical grades into the present structure, and that flexibility will be important. However, as Silver (1980) maintains, if the career structure is to establish a way in which clinical nurses can achieve financial recognition in keeping with those who pursue management or teaching, two higher levels than the existing senior grade (i.e. sister/charge nurse) should emerge.

To convey a representation of the proposed consultant in clinical nursing adequately, more detailed discussion is pursued in the next three chapters.

> The primary commitment to society of the profession of nursing
> is the practice of nursing; all other functions are secondary to it.
> (H. Peplau, *Specialisation in Nursing*)

That there is a need for the establishment of units within health care systems where 'nursing is the chief therapy, and the nurse is the chief therapist' (Tiffany, 1977) is the premise on which the whole of this book is based.

Henderson (1966) suggests that there are many situations where nursing is the only known therapy; a multidisciplinary team examining the nursing home concept identifies a need for the provision of units catering for those who need nursing care only (DHSS, 1980); Batchelor (1980) foresees a move within the British NHS to establish nursing homes where clinical charge is vested in a nurse.

Henderson (1966), in depicting total health care in the form of a pie graph, notes how different-sized 'wedges' can be seen to be appropriate to different health workers, according to the specific needs of the patient, at a given point of time. She contends that 'in some situations certain members of the team have no part of the pie, and the wedge must differ in size for each member according to the problem facing the patient, his ability to help himself, and whoever is available to help him.' The pie charts which she presents easily identify a situation in which nursing is the chief therapy (Fig. 3), and one where medicine is central (Fig. 4).

Henderson (1966) goes on to emphasise how this may change, perhaps when the woman in the body cast is discharged, and her family take on the major role, or when the young man having an amputation recovers from the operation, and the nurse takes on the major role.

A number of writers have developed the implications inherent in the second example of the young amputee. Hall (1963, 1964, 1966, 1969), Alfano (1969, 1971), Poirer (1975)

25

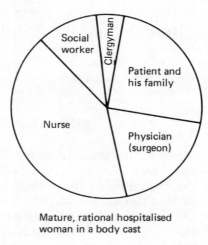

Mature, rational hospitalised
woman in a body cast

Fig. 3 Condition in which the nurse plays a major role.

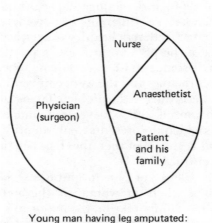

Young man having leg amputated:
day of operation

Fig. 4 Condition in which the physician plays a major role.

and Schaffrath (1978) all purport that as a patient receives medical care in response to a biological crisis, and the crisis is lessened, the intensity of medical and nursing care declines. They assert that it is at that point that the intensity of nursing should increase, as the patient's primary need becomes one for nursing care and teaching, and the need for medical care becomes less central.

Thus, many patients require care which is focused on nursing. This is not to say that their care is restricted exclusively to that of nursing, but simply that it becomes the chief therapeutic mode. Currently, the areas of long-term care for the chronically ill and elderly debilitated, and the intermediate care for those who have passed through the stage of biological crises, are the areas where nursing must take the central role. There is a tacit agreement that, in the areas of long-term care (and in the provision of community services), decision making should be undertaken by a multidisciplinary team of which the nurse is part (HMSO, 1971, 1972; British Geriatrics Society, 1976). There is now a requirement for nursing to point out where the patient's needs are essentially nursing, and where nursing care is the central component, to establish nursing as the potential leader of the team. As far as intermediate care of patients who have experienced an acute episode of illness or a breakdown in the activities of living at home, where nursing can be the major therapeutic agent to facilitate a return to maximum potential, is concerned, no provision exists within the British National Health Service, or in most Western countries.

The provision of this latter service is seen as the function of the CNU, working in co-operation with nursing home and hospital care settings.

Hall (1975) says 'Nursing home care is indicated when the primary need of the patient and his family is for a permanent home placement where care and supervision are available as needed to maintain a state of rehabilitation which the patient's maximal potential allows.' The need for this kind of care is becoming more and more apparent, particularly for the elderly. Many who live in old people's homes are too frail and dependent to be there, and equally as many occupy beds

27

in hospitals who do not require the expensive medical and ancillary services there (DHSS, 1980). There is now an increasing realisation that the provision of units where long-term patients can be cared for by professional nurses, calling in medical and other personnel as need arises, is an urgent need. Such a unit would provide care at a higher level than existing residential homes, whilst at a lesser level of sophistication than hospital care and, more importantly, based on a model for caring rather than a medical model. In this way, resources will be used wisely, and there will also be the opportunity for nursing itself to expand the nursing role. Full professional nursing practice may evolve, with nurses being accountable for the care they give, and accepting 'the responsibility without looking "up the line" for direction, or across to other disciplines, such as medicine for cover', which the Royal College of Nursing (1981) sees as the crux on which the development of true professionalism depends. Should state nursing homes emerge, the chance for the creative expansion of the nursing role may contribute greatly to the creation of nursing theory, and thus benefit all aspects of clinical nursing in all settings.

The concept of the CNU, although closely allied to the underlying principles of nursing homes (i.e. in that nursing is the major contributor to care), is seen as a separate issue. Whereas the nursing home meets the need for a permanent home placement, the CNU is seen as an attempt to provide care when the primary need of the patient and his family is for nursing care in a unit temporarily as a means of achieving recovery and return to the home environment or, when this is not possible, to placement in a nursing home. Such a unit exists in the USA, having been established as long ago as 1963 (Hall, 1964), and has been seen, on evaluation, to have had observable favourable outcomes (Hall *et al.*, 1975). The philosophy, operation and progress of this unit (the Loeb Centre for Nursing) have been well documented, yet a review of the literature by this writer has not elucidated any references to the existence of a similar unit either in the USA or Britain.

Nayer (1980) describes two 'centres of nursing excellence'

established in the USA at Rush University and Rochester University, in medical centres where nurses work largely in collaborative settings, but where new roles, especially related to extension, are developing. Both were set up in 1972, and are based on the ideal of the unification of nursing service, education, and research. Whilst the CNU postulated in this book is concerned with the care of those whose major need is nursing, and sees the purpose of such a unit as primarily development of practice, the underlying beliefs of the two centres described by Nayer can be easily extrapolated to the CNU, which is also seen as a centre of excellence.

Christman (1980b) sees the purpose of the Rush University centre, with which he is involved, as being to bridge the separation of education and service, by the use of practitioner/teachers. This, he says, will lead to:

the best prepared and most experienced nurses being available to the patient;
giving students and newly qualified nurses better behavioural models;
a greater dissemination of knowledge.

As a centre of excellence, the quality of care, educational programmes, clinical research activity, and opportunities for staff development are aimed at being notably superior to those in other centres (Christman, 1978b), and the major means used to achieve this is to keep highly qualified nurses in contact with the patient. This is, says Christman (1978a), a reversal of current trends, where 'Salary rewards are inversely related to closeness with patients'.

The centre at Rochester is based on similar beliefs, with the primary aim there being the development of 'academic leadership which exemplifies the highest standards of scholarship and clinical practice' (Ford, 1980).

Both centres embody principles suggested in this book in relation to the proposed CNU: practitioners as teachers; the need for the use of research findings and active clinical research; the need to operate as a demonstration unit; quality assurance programmes; and the need to emphasise clinical practice and autonomy and responsibility through primary nursing.

It is proposed that the CNU postulated in this book should be based on the principles adopted by the Loeb Centre for Nursing (Hall, 1964), embodying the broad beliefs on nursing held by the Rochester and Rush centres (Nayer, 1980).

Detailed and specific descriptions of setting up such a unit fall outside of the remit of this book. However, it is necessary to outline the basic principles on which the CNU may be based.

The unit itself

The CNU differs from the traditionally accepted concepts of hospitals, nursing homes, and convalescent homes. The hospital is indicated when the patient's primary need is for 'intensive medical care around the clock in conjunction with nursing care and ancillary services' (Hall, 1964). The nursing home is indicated when the primary need is for a permanent home with nursing support. The convalescent home is indicated when the patient is 'to all intents and purposes, recovered from his illness but is not believed to be strong enough to return to the pressures of his daily living' (Hall, 1964). In all of these settings, nursing is either secondary to medicine or concentrates on caretaking, rather than being the major therapy and concentrating on the healing aspect of nursing facilitated by active, dynamic and professional nursing (Alfano, 1971).

The clinical nursing unit is indicated when the patient's 'primary need is for professional nursing around the clock in conjunction with medical care and ancillary services' (Hall, 1964). The crucial implication of this is that the nurse serves as 'the chief therapist . . . working *with* the physician and other medical disciplines' (Tiffany, 1977). Although, in some cases, medical care may still be essential, nursing care is the major therapy in meeting the patient's needs for 'support, nurturing (and for) understanding his own progress and his part in it. These are the roles of nursing' (Leone, 1962). Tiffany (1977) says that 'the patient and his concerns become the focus of the process of nursing, and nursing is no longer subservient to medicine'. Drawing from the concepts inherent in the literature pertaining to the Loeb Centre for Nursing, it is possible to outline a framework to describe a CNU. Henderson (1964), in describing the newly set up centre for nursing in the USA, commented 'There *is* something new under the sun — a centre for nursing!' The idea is 'new' to nursing, and a specific and detailed description of how a CNU can be integrated into a health division or district is a task which must be approached carefully, involving representatives from the spectrum of all nursing groups and other health professionals. The discussion here is limited to the basic concepts which must be embraced in formulating plans.

The proposed clinical nursing unit serves to promote high quality nursing and, in doing so, the development of clinical nursing as a discipline through its practice, education and research. Its activities focus on nursing as a therapeutic agent — an assumption which fundamentally affirms the uniqueness of the unit. Alfano (1971) discusses nursing within the contexts of 'caretaking or healing'; although the nurse is concerned with care, Alfano asserts that 'caretaking' alone is less than professional nursing practice. She says 'If we speak of caretakers, we are talking about those who safeguard and maintain but do not initiate or change. If we speak of healers, we are talking about those who are engaged in reversing a process, that is, bringing about an acceptable change in addition to safeguarding.' Caretaking is passive and static, whereas healing is active and dynamic. The practice of nursing in the clinical nursing unit must be based on the healing potentials embodied in the acts of nursing. Hall *et al*. (1975) see the caretaking approach as being based on task-orientated practice, and the healing approach on professional-orientated practice. They demonstrate the difference between the two approaches by a list of comparative examples (Table 1). The CNU aims at professional-orientated practice, and the unit's nurses are to be charged with the task of providing 'healing' nursing.

Table 1 Comparison of task-orientated and professional-orientated practice (after Hall *et al.*, 1975)

Task-orientated practice	Professional-orientated practice
Looks upon intimate bodily care as a technical measure to produce comfort, and modifies in the light of pathology	Looks upon the comforting components of intimate bodily care and the closeness this engenders as an opportunity for nurturing, i.e. fostering growth, healing, learning, and modifies in relation to patients' concerns, feelings, as well as pathology
Therefore delegates major portion of tasks related to intimate bodily care to non-professional personnel who are least prepared to utilise the closeness in a teaching/learning situation. May or may not supervise personnel engaged in these tasks. Gives intimate bodily care only to sickest	Therefore performs all comforting measures related to intimate bodily care – delegates only work with *things* to non-professional personnel, thus freeing nurses to work with people

Admission to the clinical nursing unit

The purpose of a nursing unit is to provide care for those who need professional nursing. Referral of patients will largely be by doctors, as the need for intensive medical care rules out admission to the unit, and medical assessment must preclude this need. Clinical nurse specialists, health visitors, district nurses and others may effect referral of patients should they identify specific nursing problems, but may need to channel the referral through the patient's own doctor for medical assessment. It is anticipated that the majority of referrals will be from doctors in the acute hospital setting, or from GPs in the community, and the reason for referral must be the need for 'healing' nursing care.

In the acute hospital setting, Hall (1963) and Alfano (1969) maintain that as the need for intense medical care falls, the need for nursing rises. 'When a patient is in biological crises, the chief concern is usually whether he will live or die. As the threat of death becomes less imminent, he becomes more actively involved in working through practices associated with regaining health and re-entering the world of active community living.' (Alfano, 1969). It is at this point that referral to the CNU may be desirable.

In the community health setting, patients with nursing needs should primarily be cared for by the community services attached to the GP. Community nurses provide professional nursing services on a part-time basis to supplement the major portion of care which is given by family members. When the community nurse, and then the GP on consultation, identify problems which may be alleviated by providing full-time professional nursing on a temporary basis, to allow for re-entering the patient's own home, referral may be made to the CNU. The aim of the CNU for such admissions, from the time they enter the unit, is to help the patient to reach his maximum potential in order to return home, and the family members or other people of significance are focused on, as well as the patient, in the nursing plan. As relatives become ready, they are helped to prepare for the patient's return home, and to master any relevant activities which they may need to carry out in his care, through teaching and demonstration.

Hall (1964) outlines specific criteria for admission to the nursing unit. The patient must: be over 16 years of age (unless paediatric provision is made); require intensive nursing care in the intermediate setting (i.e. between hospital and home); be recommended by his own doctor (hospital consultant or GP); be likely to be able to return to his own community; and be expected to stay in the unit for at least one week. She suggests that the following must rule out admission to the unit.

1. The patient's return to the community is considered a physical, emotional or social improbability. (If this is the case, nursing home care is indicated.)

2. The patient can return to the community directly from the hospital under an organised home care programme (i.e. district nursing services, etc.)

3. The patient can return to the community directly from the hospital under his own family auspices.

4. The patient requires intensive medical care and diagnostic work-ups. (If this is the case, hospital admission is indicated.)

5. The patient constitutes a hazard to the safety and health of others and requires special precautionary measures.

6. The patient is eligible for transfer to existing hospital facilities for longer term care such as for tuberculosis, rehabilitation, geriatrics, etc.

Hall (1964) emphasises that the medical diagnosis of the patient is of less importance than his need for nursing.

Patients meeting the criteria would be referred by the doctor to the consultant in clinical nursing, who would undertake a nursing assessment prior to discussing the patient with the unit admission team comprising the doctor(s) attached to the unit, the social worker, and other staff members when needed (Henderson, 1964), and a decision would then be made. Discharge home would be on the basis of the achievement of nursing objectives, the feelings of the patient and his family, and discussion with the community nursing services.

With some patients, it may become apparent that they will no longer benefit from the CNU's programme, but are still unable to manage at home. In such cases, after being brought to the highest level of function, the CNU would arrange transfer to a nursing home, residential home or long-stay ward. Similarly, should the patient develop a condition which necessitates a need for high level medical care, he would be transferred to a hospital.

The unit staff

The staff of the unit would consist of the consultant in clinical nursing, professional nurses, auxilliaries, and ancillary personnel. In addition, the professional services of a doctor, physiotherapist, occupational therapist, social worker, health visitor, and community nurse would be available.

The consultant in clinical nursing is considered in Chapter 2. She is the director of the CNU and acts as leader of the team, with teaching, research and consulting functions to members of the team and those in the wider health division or district. In addition, she will have direct patient care responsibilities for her assigned patients. Harrington and Theis (1968) see the major difference between the nursing unit and other health care units lying in the fact that the 'administrative director is a professional nurse who is in charge of all the functions of the facility'.

Hall *et al*. (1975) advocate that only professional nurses should be involved in direct patient care, and that non-professional assistants should be employed to organise the 'things' needed by nurses to care for patients. Thus, auxilliaries may prepare equipment, make empty beds and help the nurse to lift. Each one of the unit's professional nurses may then act as a professional in giving direct, comprehensive nursing, being accountable for her own actions. She will not be 'the surrogate of the physician and other ancillary personnel but the surrogate of the patient' (Tiffany 1977). The organisation of care delivery is considered in Chapter 5. Essentially, each nurse in the unit, including the consultant in clinical nursing, will act as primary nurse to a group of patients, delegating care to an associate when off duty. The primary and associate nurses for a patient are the chief therapeutic agents, and the final effectors in providing inter-related patient care (Hall, 1963). Medicine and its allied professions offer ancillary help. Because all disciplines act in a consulting capacity to nursing, the nurse integrates all of her patients' therapies (Henderson, 1964).

The medical attachment to the unit may be a physician, a GP, or a group of GPs. The medical programme essentially needs to follow a pattern less like that of the hospital, and more like that of community medicine. Hall (1964) sees the unit doctor as being administratively responsible to the head of the unit, and professionally as one of a team of equals. She suggests that the medical care programme should have three main aims:

1. to evaluate the therapeutic medical plan;
2. to amend the plan when needed;
3. to add to the plan in terms of prevention, early recogni-

tion, and care of medical conditions other than those for which the patient is already receiving treatment.

The unit doctor(s) would operate much like a GP, visiting patients as need be for surveillance, and as a consultant for nurses.

The physiotherapist, other therapists, nurse specialists, etc. may act largely as resource persons to nurses, giving direct care only when special skills beyond the competencies of the nurse are demanded. Hall *et al.*'s (1975) example of the relationship between these workers and nurses, as determined by whether or not the nurse is task orientated or professional orientated, clarifies how therapists and specialists can contribute to the CNU (Table 2).

Table 2 Comparison of contributions from task-orientated and professional-orientated nurses (after Hall *et al.*, 1975)

Task-orientated practice	*Professional-orientated practice*
Other therapists (e.g. physical therapist, occupational therapist) give their care directly to patients. Nurse acts as scheduler and has little opportunity to incorporate off-floor activities into patient's activities for daily living or on-floor care	Other therapists (e.g. physical therapist, occupational therapist) act as resource persons to nurses in majority of situations – give direct care only when it is inappropriate to nursing and calls for their most distinctive area of practice. Nurses act as 'final effector'. Nurse incorporates suggestions by other therapists in her daily nursing care

Obviously, full usual supporting staff for domestic and clerical services will also be required.

The clinical nursing unit in action

It can be concluded that the CNU concept is largely one of a 'halfway house on the road to home' (Henderson, 1964) from hospital, or of an intermediate unit for the nursing rehabilitation of patients in the community who require teaching (of the patient and/or family) and nurturing to enable them to be restored to a satisfactory home life. It is feasible that it may also be used by long-term care units for patients with specific nursing problems, whereby the patient is admitted to the CNU, the problem alleviated, and then returned back to the long-term unit.

It is probable that the majority of admissions would be from acute hospital units. Henderson (1964) and Hall (1964) stress that the medical label ascribed to the patient is not of primary importance, and thus patients from the whole spectrum of medical specialities may be accommodated. Clinical nurse specialists and district nurses may utilise the CNU for the rehabilitation of patients, such as those with diabetes or colostomies, and they may wish to be attached to the unit as their patient's primary nurse in such situations. The CNU must be flexible and creative enough to encourage this kind of innovation. Patients who have overcome the biological crises of any medical condition (e.g. congestive heart failure, myocardial infarction, enucleation, orthopaedic conditions, etc.) may all benefit from admission to the CNU. Evaluation of the Loeb Centre for Nursing (Hall *et al.*, 1975) shows that the length of total stay can be shortened, the patient's quality of life at home improved, and the need for re-admission reduced, when patients are transferred to the nursing unit early after the resolution of biological crises in the hospital ward, rather than being left on the acute ward for the whole in-patient stay.

The CNU does not set out to propose that present-day nursing care in hospitals is to be devalued; nor does it intend to duplicate the activities of other units. Hospital wards are needed when biological crises arise, nursing homes when home-type care is needed, convalescent homes when the patient has no nursing problems but merely needs rest. Similarly, rehabilitation units are needed when the primary patient need is for intense physiotherapy and occupational therapy, and psychiatric wards when the primary needs are psychological. The CNU is needed when the primary need is 'teaching, counselling and nurturing which are inherent in professional nursing' (Hall, 1964).

The nursing unit emphasises nursing, whilst not devaluing the contribution of other health workers. It still collaborates with medicine, but 'nurses help patients to clarify their own goals and whatever concerns they may have with the treatment plan the physician has outlined; the nurse interprets the patient to the physician, not the physician to the patient, as in the typical hospital setting where the nurse persuades the patient that "the doctor knows best".' (Tiffany, 1977).

Can such a unit become part of our reality? Indeed, is it desirable that it should? It would seem that such a move would help in the current drive to raise the quality of nursing care, and to develop clinical nursing as a whole, Doubtlessly, because it questions the traditional structure of health care delivery, and to some extent challenges the power structure embodied in it, establishing units devoted to nursing may be opposed by some, and seen by some as simply another vehicle to achieve full professionalisation. The Academy of Nursing (1975) in the USA suggests that, if nurses 'align themselves with consumers, become politically and economically motivated, and most of all, share decision making within the health care system, patients as well as nurses will benefit.' If those involved in creating nursing units are motivated by a desire to improve patient care through professionalism, then that may well be the result, rather than solely a benefit to nursing.

The description of a CNU, and the consultant in clinical nursing role to accompany it, demands much thoughtful planning, at a much deeper and wider level than that possible in this book. However, a creative attempt to do so may have far-reaching effects on nursing care, and on the development of clinical nursing as a discipline through the generation of theory. Perhaps nursing needs people with the 'divine madness' referred to by Hall (1964) which initiates innovation, before projects such as that in the USA will be replicated in this country.

Nursing in the Clinical Nursing Unit: a Model on which to Base Nursing Practice

'But "glory" doesn't mean "a nice knockdown argument",' Alice objected.

'When I use the word', Humpty Dumpty said, in rather a scornful tone, 'it means just what I choose it to mean — neither more nor less.'

'The question is,' said Alice, 'whether you can make words mean so many different things.'

'The question is,' said Humpty Dumpty, 'which is to be master — that's all.'

(Lewis Carroll, *Through the Looking Glass*)

If the concept of a CNU, led by a consultant in clinical nursing, is accepted, then its future will depend on how well its purposes of delivering high quality nursing to those who need it and disseminating knowledge of its activities around the health district to develop the practice of clinical nursing are achieved. To fulfil these purposes, the unit must develop practice, and create an environment in which other clinical nurses can develop by experiencing the unit's activities, thus serving as a 'model' nursing unit for the health district. This chapter explores this theme by discussing nursing practice in the unit in relation to a conceptual model on which it is based.

Conceptual models

The practice of nursing within the CNU must be based on a commonly shared, basic philosophy, and utilise an agreed upon conceptual framework. Whilst the development of an appropriate conceptual framework on which to base practice for each individual nurse may well be a very individualised activity — according to Carnevali (1973) 'one that each person must do for himself' — it is useful to establish within any nursing setting a broad idea of what nursing is, what basic theories make it what it is seen to be, and in what way nursing is achieved. In other words, a shared adoption of a conceptual model for nursing practice within the CNU is advocated, and the model chosen may subsequently be modified, expanded and developed as a result of research activity in the unit generating new concepts and theories. A general concept held by the individual nurses in the unit, and shared by the group as a whole, will affect how the knowledge of nursing will be structured, and the way in which it will be applied in the practice situation.

The discussion of concepts, conceptual models, and theories of nursing is one which is plagued with confusion — and often confirms one's own doubts about intellectual capacity! McFarlane (1976) comments on the 'utter semantic confusion' in theorising in nursing, suggesting that it is 'doubtful if clarity can be restored'. Citing Dickoff and James (1968), she observes that nursing grasps at 'concrete, structural security too soon', and asserts that 'like the world of the infant, the world of theory in nursing seems a "blooming, buzzing confusion".'

This chapter attempts to explore the relevance of conceptual models to the work of the CNU, by defining the terms themselves, relating them to theories and outlining currently described conceptual models for nursing practice. The model for nursing, based on a model of living described by Roper (1976, 1979) and Roper *et al.* (1980), is then briefly explored, linking it to Orem's (1980) and Henderson's (1966) concepts, and an argument developed to support the suggestion that the utilisation of such an approach is one of choice for the CNU. If CNUs ever become a part of nursing reality, the choice of model on which to base practice will vary from unit to unit, and this, indeed, should be the case. As nursing develops, some units may begin by creating a model themselves based on concepts and theories generated within them. However, in an attempt to apply the abstract to the concrete, the model most meaningful to this writer is used as a basis for the CNU's practice of nursing.

Conceptual models and the practice of nursing

McFarlane (1976) purports that 'the registered nurse must practise from a theoretical basis adequate to her function if the care she gives is to be safe and of good quality. At any level of skill in nursing, the practitioner needs a basis of theory adequate to support practice at that level.' What, then, is theory? Riehl and Roy (1980) define a theory as 'a scientifically acceptable principle which governs practice or is proposed to explain observable facts . . . a logically interconnected set of propositions used to describe, explain, or predict a part of the empirical world.' The *Kings English Dictionary* (1930) says a theory is 'a doctrine, or scheme of things, which terminates in speculation or contemplation without a view to practice; an exposition of the general principles of any science; the philosophical explanation of phenomena, either physical or moral.' Riehl and Roy thus see theory as governing practice; the *Kings English Dictionary* sees it as principles when related to science, and thus having implications on the application of science. Nursing theory is defined by Riehl and Roy (1980) as a 'conceptual structure of knowledge useful and necessary to attain the goals established by nurses'.

Theory is built up from concepts, and a concept is 'an abstract general notion' (*Kings English Dictionary*, 1930). Hardy (1973) describes how concepts and theories relate: 'Concepts are labels, categories, or selected properties of objects to be studied; they are the bricks from which theories are constructed . . . concepts are the basic elements of theory.' McFarlane (1976) suggests that nursing is still at the stage of concept identification rather than theory formulation, and points out that the multitude of concepts already identified in nursing indicate how complex nursing is. She foresees the development of a range of theories of nursing rather than a single, unitary theory. Concepts of nursing are being identified by many nurse writers, particularly in North America (e.g. Riehl and Roy, 1980), and more may emerge from the diverse settings in which nursing takes place, and as nurses increasingly strive for a theoretical basis for their practice. Rines and Montag (1976) say that concepts are representations of ideas which can serve as guides. Nursing theories can either select relevant, guiding concepts from other bodies of knowledge, e.g. physiology, psychology etc. — a method referred to as deductive theory building — or develop new nursing concepts by analysing current nursing practice, which is inductive theory building. Deductive theory building begins with general concepts and applies the general to the specific, whereas the inductive method begins with the specific and then generalises. It has been suggested that inductive theory building in nursing begins with 'practical nursing experience' and develops concepts by the 'inductive analysis of this experience rather than borrowing concepts that they feel will fit'. McFarlane (1976) proposes that both methods must be utilised for nursing theory to be developed, whilst emphasising that theory for nursing grows out of the practice of nursing.

Comments made by Dickoff and James on theory in nursing point out the relationship between the activities of the CNU and the identification of concepts and theories: 'We need to ask "What's the use of theory? Why bother to theorise and to research?" Our contention is that nursing practice is the alpha and omega of nursing theorising and nursing research. The impetus for nursing theorising and researching must arise from practice, since nursing is a practice.' Alongside the present approaches to theorising and research— i.e. academics, senior managers and educators conducting research in nursing settings which they choose and work in as researchers, and creating theory away from the clinical scene — the CNU nurses will approach them from a stance which is firmly rooted in clinical nursing practice.

Concepts and theories may be utilised to create a conceptual model for nursing practice. The term 'model' is defined by Riehl and Roy (1980) as 'a construct related to theory', and by McFarlane (1976) as 'a conceptual representation of reality'. Johnson (1980) describes a conceptual model for nursing practice as 'a systematically constructed, scientifically based, and logically related set of concepts which identify the essential components of nursing practice together with the values required in their use by the practitioner'. This 'diagram' of what nursing practice is, provides for the nurse, according to Riehl and Roy (1980), a diagnostic and treatment orientation for the specific practice of nursing. It provides the unifying framework for an organised way of looking at nursing. Roper (1976) maintains that it is impossible to define nursing satisfactorily in a way which fits every setting, and that the only way in which nursing can be described is by constructing a conceptual model. Models provide blueprints for the application of theory to the seeker of nursing, by the giver of nursing, and thus serve as sound guidelines for nursing practice.

Until recent years, and in many parts of the world now, nursing had been practised from the basis of disease/medical/hospital-orientated models. Contemporary nursing is developing its own models, based primarily on interactionist, systems, and developmental theories (Riehl and Roy, 1980). Using the nursing process as a means to deliver nursing care, nurses use a conceptual model on which to base assessment, problem identification, care planning, implementation of care, and evaluation of the outcomes. Orem (1980) suggests that if nurses use the concepts and theories inherent in a conceptual model for nursing practice, they will practise more effectively, and will be able to 'place in perspective, other descriptions of nursing including those in areas of nursing specialisation'. Thus she, along with Roper (1976), believes that a satisfactory model will describe nursing in any context: it will have meaning to nurses in all of the medical specialties, specialties arising from classifications of age groups (e.g. paediatrics), and specialties determined by the setting in which care is given (e.g. community nursing). Orem (1980) goes on to observe that, through the emergence of models specifically for nursing, the nurse's role is 'emerging from obscurity imposed by an over-emphasis on the relationship between the physician and the nurse, and between the employing institution and the nurse . . . Nurses are coming to recognise that an item of information about a patient may have one meaning for a physician, but quite a different meaning for the nurse.' Conceptual models may thus be seen as a starting point to developing the professional practice of clinical nursing — an aspiration of the CNU.

A number of conceptual models are described in the literature (Roper, 1979; Blake, 1980; Chrisman and Fowler, 1980; Johnson, 1980; Neuman, 1980; Orem, 1980; Riehl, 1980; Roy 1980), and an attempt is made by Riehl and Roy (1980) to construct a unified model for nursing by amalgamating a variety of models. It is useful to view models as sources of guidance, each one having overlapping similarities, and to accept the possibility of adopting one model of choice whilst also borrowing concepts from others to form a meaningful base for practice. Regardless of the theory used, the nursing process can be utilised to implement practice based on a specific model.

The division of types of models into systems, developmental and interactionist frameworks, described by Riehl and Roy (1980), is useful in discussing currently described models.

Systems models are derived from predictions based on scientific principles. Neuman's (1980) model, for example, focuses on stress — how the patient responds to it and how nursing can help — whilst Roy's (1980) model focuses on adaptation to changes arising in the area of physiological needs, self-concept, role function and interdependency. Orem's (1980) model concentrates on man's need for self-care action and the 'provision and management of it' by nursing (Calley *et al.*, 1980; Coleman, 1980).

Developmental models emphasise how the patient evolves with a past, present and future, and identify the variables which the nurse is aware of in nursing the patient. They centre on growth and directional change, thus assuming that change is the focus of nursing (Chin, 1980). Peplau's (1969) model focuses on the growth of the patient and the nurse, emphasising the phases and roles through which both pass in the interpersonal process. Travelbee's (1971) model has a similar emphasis, whilst the developmental model described by Chrisman and Fowler (1980) focuses on the continuous change process in biological, social and personal systems.

Interactionist models centre upon what transpires between the nurse and the patient's 'interpersonal lifestyle', and the theory of symbolic interactionism. Riehl's (1980) model focuses on symbolic interactionism in the nurse–patient relationship, and the role of the nurse as patient advocate.

Riehl and Roy (1980) argue that the theorists who devise models view man similarly, and that a unified model for nursing may be a desirable aim. Though details within specific models vary from one to the other, most nursing models are more similar to each other than different, and unifying these models into a theoretical amalgam may allow for a common structure for nursing practice. McFarlane (1976) hopes for a multiplicity of theoretical models, and thus conceptual models, and finds the idea of a unitary theory for nursing impracticable and untenable. She proclaims 'Let us beware of grasping any structural security which is not reflected in the reality of nursing practice; let us rather have the courage to fumble a little longer isolating concepts, testing hypotheses. Building theories may never again be so exciting as it is for us who are at the beginning of such an exercise.'

The task of the CNU is to choose a conceptual model on which to base practice, and evaluate, develop, and change it in the practical reality of a setting where nursing is taking place. In doing so, the value of operating from a conceptual framework may be established and disseminated around the health district served by the CNU. The choice of a model is dependent on the consultant in clinical nursing and the unit staff, and the model to be discussed here is selected essentially according to the biases and beliefs of this writer.

Roper (1976 and 1979), and Roper *et al.* (1980) describe a systems/development-based model for nursing, which incorporates many of the concepts inherent in the model described by Orem (1980) and the conceptual framework presented by Henderson (1966). The model for nursing is based on a model of living, and attempts to identify a concept of nursing to help nurses to develop a mode of thinking about nursing centred on the process of living. The Nursing Developmental Conference Group (1973) purports that a concept of the reality of nursing is the only basis from which it can progress. A concept of nursing is needed for the CNU to organise nursing reality and to look at theory differently in the fields of theory building and research and prac-

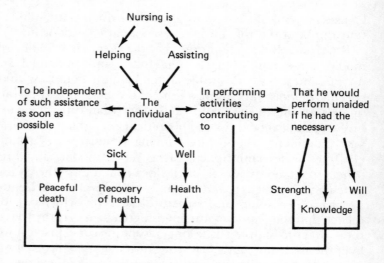

Fig. 5 A concept of nursing constructed from Henderson's (1966) concepts (NDCG, 1975).

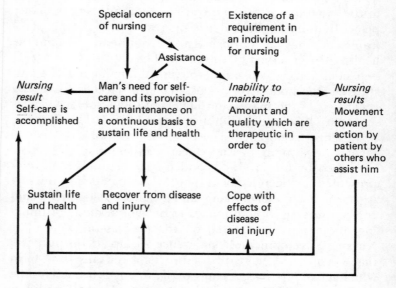

Fig. 6 A concept of nursing constructed from Orem's (1980) concepts (NDCG, 1975).

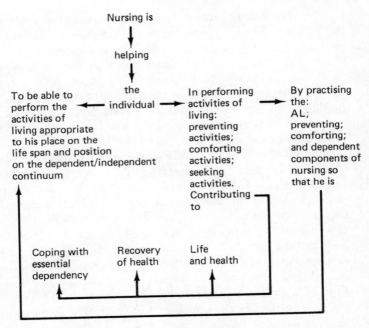

Fig. 7 A concept of nursing constructed from Roper *et al.*'s (1980) concepts.

tice. A concept of nursing identifies the elements and relation-ships upon which the nurse can focus in nursing situations. The NDCG (1973) examines the concepts of various theorists, and organises them to present an overall concept of nursing for each. The concepts of nursing attributable to Henderson (1966) and Orem (1980) are in Figs. 5 and 6 respectively; and, using the same approach as the NDCG, an attempt to organise the concept of Roper *et al.* (1980) appears in Fig. 7. The similarities between the three approaches are evident.

The model for nursing based on a model of living was developed from the findings of a research study into clinical experience for student nurses (Roper, 1976). Roper (1976) describes the purpose of the model as the promotion of the development of nursing as a discipline. Wilson (1972) pur-ports that disciplines are 'forms of thought that have a characteristic approach to appropriate questions related to the subject'. Roper (1976) suggests that the use of a conceptual model will allow nurses to think 'nursologically' — i.e. in a way characteristic of nursing, much in the same way as mathematicians think mathematically, theologians theologically, and anatomists anatomically. She asserts that her model is 'an attempt to initiate a conceptual structure for nursing which could be used as a base from which the discipline of nursing could develop'.

Roper *et al.*'s (1980) model for nursing identifies the subject of nursing as the individual, seeing him as a person engaged in living through his life span. Related to, but not entirely dependent on, the life span is a dependent/independent continuum, the individual moving towards each end of the continuum dynamically depending upon the developmental stages of the life span, and immediate circumstances such as environment, state of health, etc. In living, the individual partakes of, or requires help with, four groups of activities, all four of which are interrelated, and are only divided into discrete entities for the purpose of analysis. The four groups of activities are:

activites of living;
preventing activities;
comforting activities;
seeking activities.

From all of these concepts, a model of living is constructed (Table 3).

Although all four groups of activities are so interrelated that in reality they cannot be seen to be separate, it is useful to discuss their essence separately.

Activities of living

Most people engage in the full range of these activities in their daily life. However, there are stages in the life span when the individual cannot yet, or can no longer, perform one or more

48

Table 3 A model of living

Activities of living	Life span		
	Conception ⟶ Death		
Preventing	Continuum		
Comforting	Totally dependent ⟷ Totally independent		
Seeking			
Maintaining a safe environment	_____		
Communicating	_____		
Breathing	_____		
Eating and drinking	_____		
Eliminating	_____		
Personal cleansing and dressing	_____		
Controlling body temperature	_____		
Mobilising	_____		
Working and playing	_____		
Expressing sexuality	_____		
Sleeping	_____		
Dying	_____		

of the activities, and specific circumstances may restrict performance in one or more activity. Thus, there are times in the life span when the individual is at a point nearer to the dependent or independent pole of the dependence/independence continuum, and movement along the continuum is dynamic. Performance of the activities of living (ALs) involves the three other groups of activities, so that preventing, seeking and comforting activities are all involved with:

maintaining a safe environment
communicating
breathing
eating and drinking
eliminating

personal cleansing and dressing
controlling body temperature
mobilising
working and playing
expressing sexuality
sleeping
dying.

Preventing activities

These are the activities in which individuals engage to prevent those things which will impair living, such as illness and accidents. They include a vast array of almost unconscious acts performed as a result of socialisation. Performing personal hygiene to prevent infection, and following road rules to prevent accidents are examples of preventing activities.

Comforting activities

These are the activities which a person performs to give physical, psychological and social comfort. A person who is suffering from a common cold, who rests in bed, keeps warm, etc. is an example of someone engaging in comforting activities.

Seeking activities

These are the activities in which the person engages in the pursuit of knowledge, new experience, and answers to novel problems. The person who goes to a doctor because he is ill is engaging in a seeking activity.

Roper (1976) emphasises the closeness and overlapping of the four groups of activities. If a person is suffering from extreme headaches, he will, by carrying out certain *ALs, seek comfort* by consulting a doctor and thus try to overcome the condition, and *prevent* it from re-occuring.

The model of living represents the individual— the subject of nursing — engaged in the process of living. Roper (1976) describes the subject of nursing thus: 'Basically, man is

Table 4 A model for nursing

Nursing components	Patient's life span
	Conception ————▶ Death
	Totally dependent ◀——▶ Totally independent
	Circumstance

Activities of living

preventing _____

comforting _____

dependent _____

_____

_____

_____

_____

_____

_____

_____

_____

envisaged as carrying out various activities during a life span
from conception to death. His main objective is to attain self-
fulfilment and maximum independence in each activity of
daily living within the limitations set by his particular circumstances. He also carries out many activities of a preventing, comforting and seeking nature and he appropriately
alters priorities among the activities of daily living. In these
ways, the individual endeavours to be healthy and independent in the process of living.'

Using this model, Roper *et al*. (1980) develop a model for
nursing (Table 4).

Illness is seen as but an episode in the life of an individual,
and it is proposed that nursing must be approached within the
context of the patient's process of living. Nursing is based on a
model of living, and is modelled as being composed of four
components, which equate with the four groups of activities in
the model of living. The recipient of nursing is viewed within

his life span, and in relation to the dependence/independence continuum.

Activities of living component of nursing

This is the central component of nursing, and is concerned with acquiring, maintaining or restoring maximum independence for the individual, or enabling him to cope with dependency in any of the ALs should circumstances make this necessary. Nursing may need to inform, provide material resources for, or actually carry out activities for the individual.

Preventive component of nursing

This is essentially a part of every nursing activity. It includes the prevention of such things as pressure sores, dehydration, boredom etc. as well as facilitating the acquisition of relevant knowledge by the patient to prevent ill-health, through health education.

The preventive components are modelled as supporting the AL components with the objective of minimising the dependence of each patient or client (Roper, 1976).

Comforting component of nursing

This may be equated with the 'nurturing' aspect, seen by many as fundamental to nursing (Hall, 1969), or the 'art' of nursing (Roper *et al.*, 1980). It includes such things as helping the patient into a position for physical comfort, taking his hand in an offer of companionship, and placing items he needs close at hand. The comforting components of nursing are inherent in every interaction between the nurse and the patient. They are modelled as supporting the AL components with the objective of maximising the independence of each patient or client (Roper, 1976).

Dependent component of nursing

In the model of living, seeking activities are identified as one of the four groups, and the dependent component of nursing aims at meeting the goals of these activities. When a person is ill, he seeks medical help, and may need nursing. When he is unable to reach his maximum level of independence, although not ill, he may need nursing. Roper (1976) describes this component as 'medically prescribed' and comprising those tasks prescribed by the doctor, to be carried out by the nurse. For example giving medications, performing dressings, etc. This component of nursing is modelled as supporting the AL components, again with the objective of achieving maximum independence for each patient.

Operationalising the model is seen to be best effected by utilising the 'process of nursing' (Roper *et al.*, 1980). Thus, the model and the means by which it is applied can be combined to construct the model for nursing shown in Table 5. How each step in the process is carried out is greatly influenced by the concepts in the model. For example, assessment will be largely based on the individual ALs.

It is proposed that the model for nursing based on a model of living described by Roper *et al.* (1980) is the most suitable model for utilisation in a British CNU. It gives a global concept of nursing, transcending the boundaries which exist between various nursing contexts, and may be applied in all fields of nursing. It points out the knowledge base needed by all nurses, and identifies the uniqueness of nursing. Most important at this stage in the development of British clinical nursing, it speaks to nurses in a language which is familiar, and related to nursing in this country. The fact that the vast literature on conceptual models for nursing practice is written in the language of North American nurses — one which is almost incomprehensible to most British nurses— is perhaps the main reason why theories are not widely applied in current nursing practice— a point of much relevance to this discussion, and to the development of clinical nursing in Britain. Kron (1972), herself from the USA, heavily criticises the way in which the language of nursing has developed there,

Table 5 A model for nursing and the means by which it is applied

Nursing components	Patient's life span
	Conception ———▶ Death
	Totally dependent ◀——▶Totally independent
	Circumstance

Activities of living

  preventing   ————————————————————

  comforting   ————————————————————

  dependent   ————————————————————

————————————————————

————————————————————

————————————————————

————————————————————

————————————————————

————————————————————

————————————————————

————————————————————

Assessment of patient ——▶ Identification of patient's problems and
statement of expected outcomes

                       ↓
                       Planning
                       ↓
                       Implementation
                       ↓
                       Evaluation

and there is a very real need for literature able to convey
meaningful messages on conceptual models to the vast
number of practising clinical nurses in Britain. Van Dersal
(1974) describes a tool he has devised to calculate the amount
of meaning conveyed to a given audience by a given dialogue,
known as the 'fog index'. It would seem that much of the
literature on models is indeed masked by a fog to British
nurses, and it would be useful to apply the index to such
writings. Kron (1972) points out how simple words with
widely known meanings, such as 'carry out', are now being
replaced by 'jargon' words such as 'implement'. Recent

discussions with American nurses revealed a similar dissatisfaction with the new language of nursing, generating the
adoption, for example, of the term 'Oremese' to describe the
language of Orem's (1980) *Nursing: concepts of practice*. Van
Dersal's (1974) example of the misuse of language may
demonstrate how true meaning can be distorted:

> 'Ornithological specimens of identical plumage usually congregate in
> the closest possible proximity' may be used to convey the simple
> message of: 'Birds of a feather flock together'.

McFarlane (1976) says 'the purpose of a practice theory is
to be able to make a prescription for practice where, after all,
nursing begins and ends. Hence, I am often a little sceptical of
theories of nursing which seem to bear no relationship to any
practice I have ever seen.' It is not suggested here that the
models described in the literature bear no relationship to
practice — rather that they are frequently seen to bear no
relationship to British clinical nurses because of the language
usage. Roper *et al.*'s (1980) model represents the only
developed model published by and for British nurses. Its
greatest advantage, then, is its ability to convey meaning to
clinical nurses.

Having argued for the use of a specific model on which to
base the practice of the CNU, it must be said that no model
can be accepted as a final representation of reality, but only as
a basis for further analysis, concept identification, and theory
building and testing leading to a dynamic and developing
approach to the practice of nursing. As an initial spring-board
from which the CNU can dive into the task of developing
clinical practice, Roper *et al.*'s (1980) model is useful, but the
continuous re-interpretation and modification of the basis of
practice is the crucial work of the CNU. A model for practice is
broader than a concept or theory — it is constructed of them
(Riehl and Roy, 1980). In utilising a conceptual model for
practice, the CNU does not rest on its laurels, but strives to
re-shape the model towards perfection in the light of the new
knowledge generated by concept and theory building.
McFarlane (1980) purports that theories about self-care,
agency, continence, design— theories which are prescriptive

of a better quality of nursing action because they are based on a scientific framework — are urgently needed. In basing its practice on a conceptual model, the CNU must attempt to utilise or to meet these urgent needs for nursing.

5 | Organising Nursing in the Clinical Nursing Unit

> She makes me wash, they comb me all to thunder — the widder eats by a bell; she gets up by a bell — everything's so awful reg'lar a body can't stand it.
>
> (Mark Twain, *The Adventures of Tom Sawyer*)

> An unlearned carpenter of my acquaintance once said in my hearing 'There is very little difference between one man and another; but what little there is, is very important.' This seems to me to go to the root of the matter.
>
> (William James, *The Will to Believe, The Importance of Individuals*)

There is an attempt in the CNU to create an environment in which professional nursing can take place, based on a conceptual model and emphasising the essence of nursing. It is necessary to explore the various methods of giving nursing in terms of the management of care delivery.

The purpose of the CNU is the same as that defined by Kron (1976) in relation to any hospital ward — to care for the patient either directly, through actual patient care, or indirectly through research and training. The latter two are considered in Chapter 6. Sjoberg *et al.* (1971) list four factors which determine the quality of care that a nurse is able to give.

1. The ability of the nurse.
2. The physical environment.
3. The philosophy of administration.
4. The method of assignment.

The fourth factor is the area of organisation to be considered in this chapter. The emergence of task or job assignment as a method of organising nursing has been mentioned in Chapter 1 and some historical reasons for its adoption suggested. This way of delivering care to patients in hospitals is by far the most common and has been the traditional concept of nursing care for a number of years. It emphasises efficiency and division of labour, requiring rigid controls and denying the importance of psychosocial needs of patients and staff. The utilisation of a task assignment approach reflects the adoption of an administrative model of practice and militates against any achievement of professional authority (Etzioni, 1969). Economic pressures to use trained nurses efficiently, a belief in the scientific management theories (Tyler, 1965), and the historical roots of nursing have all served to promote the adoption of task assignment as a method of organising nursing, and nurse training has effectively socialised students into valuing routine and feeling satisfaction and fulfilment in the completion of tasks (Anderson, 1973; Lelean, 1973; Davies, 1976; Davies, 1977). Observation of nurses at work suggests that the major impetus in work patterns is towards completing tasks and then withdrawing from the patient area, thus avoiding patient contact (Stockwell, 1972; Hawthorn, 1974; Cleary, 1977). Such a strategy may have evolved to avoid the stress and anxiety inherent in close nurse–patient relationships, and may form part of the social defence system against anxiety in nursing suggested by Menzies (1960).

The carrying out of discrete jobs or tasks is said to fragment care, emphasise physical care, ignore psychosocial care and a holistic approach to nursing, and prevent any progression towards professional autonomy in nursing. Several studies have shown that this method prevents care which meets the individual needs of the patient (Hamilton-Smith, 1972; Wright, 1974; Hayward, 1975). In one study (Anderson, 1973), patients themselves felt that nurses failed to spend time on talking to individual patients, or answering questions. The performance of each task and the planning of treatment and care regimes based on the daily task assignments are routinised ruthlessly (Davies, 1976, 1977), and 'procedure manuals' detail specifically how each task should be performed. It seems apparent that giving nursing according to a task assignment system is not the mark of professional nursing practice, and that it does not meet the individualised, holistic needs of patients.

There is now considerable interest shown by nurses in devising methods of organising nursing to facilitate holistic care and opportunities for professional practice in its truest sense. Marram (1979) says that any method of organising nursing should aim at:

1. unifying the patient's care to minimise fragmentation;
2. placing nursing care at the patient's side to avert the pyramiding of nursing care delivery and the nurse's preoccupation with the hierarchy.

The methods of team nursing, unit assignment, and primary nursing are all attempts to achieve such objectives.

Team nursing

Kron (1976) maintains that team nursing is more of a philosophy than a method of organising nursing, and Barrett (1968), whilst agreeing, suggests that it is also a methodology for care: 'Team nursing is said to be a philosophy rather than a way of working. Perhaps it is both, for patients are assigned, and staff is organised in special ways when team nursing is practised. Yet as a philosophy, team nursing expresses beliefs about patients, personnel, leadership, and relationships.'

A team is a group of persons working together towards a common goal (*Kings English Dictionary*, 1930). A nursing team, according to Leino (1951), is a 'group of professional and non-professional nursing service personnel working together in planning, giving, and evaluating patient-centred nursing care to a group of patients'.

Team nursing aims at achieving nursing care objectives through the action of a group of nurses, and is based on a belief that participative management gives better job satisfaction and motivation (Kron, 1976). The nursing team is composed of two or more members of staff (one being designated as leader), who are assigned the care of a group of patients (Lambertson, 1953). Advocates of this method state that the team leader must be a professional, i.e. registered nurse (Leino, 1951; Lambertson, 1953; Barrett, 1968; Kron, 1976). In a ward where the number of patients is small, Barrett (1968) suggests below 15, only one nursing team may be needed, but in the more usual larger wards of 20–40 beds, two or more

59

team leaders and their teams may function under the direction of the ward sister. The team leader is delegated responsibility for providing nursing care for all patients in her assigned group. The team itself may be made up of a registered nurse leader, student or pupil nurses, and nursing auxillaries, although there is nothing in the philosophy of team nursing to preclude teams composed entirely of trained nurses. The reality of manpower resources alone dictates that this be an unattainable hope within the foreseeable future. Barrett (1968) outlines the functioning of the nursing team. The leader and team members, with the participation of the ward sister, assess, plan, implement and evaluate nursing care for each individual patient. To allow this process to occur, a daily team conference is held where care plans are reviewed, progress notes discussed, and needed changes made. The leader plans assignments of nurses to patients within the team, and supervises and informally instructs team members. Barrett (1968) sees the team conference as the 'greatest single distinguishing feature of the nursing team method of assignment. Without it, the assignment is no different from the patient or functional method except that the team leader, instead of the head nurse, delegates the duties. The heart of the team concept is group planning.'

As a method of nursing care delivery, team nursing began to be utilised in Britain some years ago (Brenham, 1971) and offers a number of advantages. As the team assigned to care for the patient is constant, the patient is able to develop relationships more easily with the carers, and continuity of care is promoted. As authority is decentralised, the team leader is given an opportunity for growth in terms of leadership skills, and supervision of unqualified staff is closer. Manthey (1970) and Marram (1979), however, are critical of it as a method to facilitate individualised nursing. The method is often misinterpreted by clinical nurses and used merely as a method of organising work rather than as a philosophy. As such, it may simply maintain a task assignment approach, on a scale smaller than when teams are not used.

Unit assignment

Sjoberg *et al*. (1971) describe a method of organising nursing based on the progressive patient care concept, calling it *Unit Assignment: a patient centred system*. Developed for a Canadian hospital setting, the method is based on findings from an extensive preliminary research study aimed at identifying the activity patterns of nurses involved in patient care, and establishing a method by which high quality patient-centred care could be provided within the existing constraints of staffing policies (Holmlund, 1967; Sjoberg, 1968; Sjoberg and Bicknell, 1969). In line with the progressive patient care concepts to which the method adheres, the research led to the development of a tool to classify patients into four care levels:

intense,
above average,
average,
minimal.

Arising from this, Sjoberg *et al*. (1971) developed the unit assignment method of organising nursing care. The ward structure is decentralised, and divided into units of care for each of the four care levels. Each small unit of care is complete in terms of equipment and facilities, and the nurse's station for each is situated close to the patients. Each day, the patient is reviewed, and placed in the unit of care corresponding to the level in which he is classified. Within each unit of care, nursing is said to be patient centred and the nursing team operates in the same way as that in team nursing.

Although this method is an efficient way to utilise nursing manpower resources, it would appear to militate against the establishment of long-term, meaningful relationships between patients and nurse, and thus continuity of care. There is a possibility that the movement of the patient from one area to another may well lead to anxiety or distress for the patient.

Primary nursing

Primary nursing is a development of the case method, which was the practice norm until the 1930s (Beyers and Phillips, 1971). In the case method, or patient allocation, one nurse performs all nursing care for patients, and thus real autonomy and the opportunity for developing a close therapeutic relationship are prevalent. However, the case method is not administratively or economically feasible for general adoption in Britain at the moment. Primary nursing is seen as a return to a case method orientation, with a primary nurse assuming responsibility for a caseload of patients throughout their hospital stay, or care by community services (Manthey, 1970). The primary nurse holds 24-hour, seven days a week responsibility for planning and administering care, though obviously only providing actual care during her hours on duty. When she is off duty, care is continued by an associate nurse (Elhart *et al.*, 1978). The associate nurse follows the care plan developed by the primary nurse, although Manthey *et al.* (1970) suggest that the associate 'may change parts of the care plan to reflect changes in the patient's condition; however, the primary nurse is responsible for any fundamental changes in the design of the plan'. Donovan (1971) points out that although primary nursing appears to demand 24-hour responsibility for the patient by the primary nurse, responsibility is delegated to associate nurses on each shift not covered by the primary nurse.

Such a system may well be feasible within the NHS in Britain and thus the CNU. If full responsibility for 24 hours a day were given to the primary nurse, then it may be assumed that there may be occasions when the associate nurse may need to contact, or even call in, the off-duty primary nurse for advice, when crucial events occur. Primary nurses may, justifiably, demand special financial arrangements to cover such eventualities, and the current financial difficulties, combined with the bureaucratic structure of health care facilities may preclude such an innovation. Thus, if 24-hour responsibility is unrealistic, Manthey's application of the primary nursing method may be the answer.

Manthey *et al*. (1970) and Manthey (1970, 1973) describe the introduction of the primary nurse method in a medical ward in the USA. Each RN and licensed practical nurse (LPN) on the ward was given primary responsibility for a group of patients numbering from three to six, and the skill of each nurse was considered in assigning her to patients. The primary nurse assesses her patient on admission, prepares a care plan, and is responsible for implementing the plan and its continuous evaluation. When she is off duty, responsibility is delegated by her to an associate. Elpern (1977) discusses the utilisation of the primary nursing approach based on geo-graphically defined units within the ward, calling it 'modular nursing'. Each module is composed of 10 to 12 patients, and nurses are permanently assigned to the module with off duties arranged so that staff within the module cover others who are off duty. The module leader has 24-hour responsibility for her patients (i.e. she is the primary nurse) and has the opportunity to move to all shifts should she wish to. This supporting arrangement for primary nursing may be useful, but may also be a compromise and may tend to become similar to a team nursing approach. The approach described by Manthey *et al*. appears to have become well accepted, and is, Manthey says, 'alive and well in the hospital' (Manthey, 1973).

The emphasis on the one-to-one, client–professional rela-tionship, and thus the facilitation of professional nursing practice, makes primary nursing the method of choice in organising nursing in the CNU. The idea of 24-hour respon-sibility, especially for the consultant in clinical nursing, is perhaps worthy of consideration. If the CNU is to act as a centre to develop and evaluate innovation in the delivery of care, and the consultant in clinical nursing is to act in a real consultant role, the constraints normally imposed on nursing by the NHS structure must be less inflexible. Thus, it may be possible for the consultant in clinical nursing, if the unit bed complement is small, to be the primary nurse for each patient, and accept 24-hour responsibility, and only delegate implementation of the care plan to an associate when off duty. Alternatively, in a larger unit, each nurse may accept 24-hour responsibility for a group of patients, and in cases where admission is initiated by a clinical nurse specialist, she may take responsibility. Wolford (1964) describes a method of assignment where one nurse plans and provides comprehensive, individualised care for patients on a 24-hour basis both before and after hospitalisation. She terms this 'complemental nursing' and sees it as a combination and refinement of the idea of care by a physician and care by a private duty nurse. The unifying of the primary nursing and complemental nursing concepts may well be the ideal method of organising care in the CNU.

In practical terms, the combination of both concepts may be applied as follows. The patient, on referral to the CNU, will be assigned to a primary nurse: this may be the consultant in clinical nursing, a unit nurse, or a clinical nurse specialist from the health district who wishes to admit a patient for specialist care. The primary nurse would then be responsible for the nursing care of the patient before, during, and after admission to the unit. She will assess, plan and evaluate care, and implement and plan when on duty. When she is off duty, implementation of the plan will be delegated to an associate, and this may be a community nurse before and after admission, or a unit nurse during the patient's stay in the unit. Should the plan require major changes when the primary nurse is off duty, or a crucial event in the patient's life requiring the presence of the primary nurse occur, the associate may call in the primary nurse. Such an approach may hold many complications, and prove impractical, but testing such an application may prove useful.

The method of organising clinical nursing has implications for the type of care provided, and for the development of clinical nursing. The most crucial determinant of how the patient is nursed, however, may lie in the philosophy of nursing held by the group of care givers, and the nursing knowledge and skill possessed. Donovan (1971) purports that the various methods of the care delivery currently being developed (e.g. team nursing, primary nursing) have had only limited success, and asks if this may be because 'the greatest emphasis and effect has been placed on the delivery system, rather than focusing primarily on nursing care'.

Whilst introducing a workable method of delivering clinical nursing and evaluating its efficacy is one aspect of the CNU's work, its greatest task still lies in the development of suitable means to provide nursing through research and innovation.

6 | Research and Teaching in the Clinical Nursing Unit

> We shall never know the answers, let alone the questions, unless we take a good, hard look at what may at first hand seem to be simple things and therefore beneath us. They are the stuff of which nursing is made. If we don't ask questions, who will?
> (Charlotte Kratz, *Those Baths . . .*)

The proposed CNU has two purposes: to provide high quality nursing to those who seek, are directed to, or need nursing; and, by doing so, to develop the practice of clinical nursing. Both of these purposes can only be realised if the delivery of nursing care by the staff of the unit is accompanied by meaningful clinical nursing research, and the teaching of unit staff and nurses within the wider health district. This is true of any setting in which nursing takes place, but the distinction here is that the research and teaching emphasis is on the reality of direct delivery of nursing in a setting where nursing is central, and research into it is embodied in the goals of the nursing team's efforts.

Research

Treece and Treece (1977) assert that nursing research has traditionally concentrated on nursing education and nursing administration, and the nurse. Although the delivery of nursing care to patients is the ultimate objective of all nurses, whether they be educators, managers or clinicians, clinical nursing research 'has been largely ignored by researchers until recently'. Abdellah and Levine (1965) observe that 'the study of nursing practice itself and the study of the art and science underlying the practice of nursing are only beginning to be recognised as "musts" for the profession.' Abdellah *et al*. (1960) emphasise a need for clinical nursing research —

research into the actual acts comprising clinical nursing rather than into the organisation of nursing, who or what nurses are, and how they learn — and regret the scarcity of clinical research emphasising the need for 'descriptive research' conducted in the 'real world' of the patient.

The CNU is seen as a centre for clinical nursing research for a health district. As such, it will educate its nurses in research methodology, utilise research findings, conduct clinical research itself, and disseminate information to nurses in the area it serves. In carrying out these activities, it is hoped that the CNU will orientate nurses to a research-based practice for nursing. The 'research mindedness' and activity of the unit may serve to improve nursing for its recipients, and develop the practice of nursing through the generation and/or validation of nursing knowledge.

Jacox (1974) purports that 'practice can only be as sound as the knowledge on which it is based'. Donovan (1971) cites Diers' belief that the essence of good nursing practice requires clinical nursing research, without which nursing is 'an empty ritual' and not thoughtful practice. The improvement of nursing practice, says Beland (1970), depends on the study of present and new practices, and she adds that 'in today's world one either goes forward or goes backward. There is no standing still.' She goes on to observe that it is possible to base activities on intuition and experience and that this has been the dictum of nursing for too long. There is now a need to establish an identifiable body of knowledge on which to base practice, and the development of such a body of knowledge is the concern of clinical research. Nursing decisions based on the knowledge of possibilities are more likely to be correct than those made according to rule, or intuitively.

Much has been said and written about the need for clinical research in nursing, and nurses are frequently exhorted to develop clinical research (Bond, 1978). In the USA, the National Committee for Study expressed a regret that 'so little research has been conducted to determine the relative effectiveness of various forms of nursing intervention, and the impact of particular innovations in nursing practice . . . We are confident that only through research can we begin to determine and fully exploit the capabilities of nurses to contribute to the health system.' This, in a country where nursing research studies proliferate to a much greater extent than in Britain. McFarlane (1980), speaking from within the British context, implies that clinical research has begun in Britain, 'but the studies in clinical nursing which have so far been undertaken are, of necessity, descriptive studies, and nursing as a practice discipline is in need of studies which will provide prescriptive data.' The Report of the Committee on Nursing (1972) recommends that 'Direct research into clinical nursing and midwifery problems, which we regard as being of great importance, should begin in the ward itself or at field level in the community. Such research has direct and obvious implications for patient care.' In a previous paragraph, they assert that 'a sense of the need for research should become part of the mental equipment of every practising nurse and midwife'.

The mammoth task of orientating nurses to this 'research mindedness' approach to practice may be accomplished, in part, by the presence, close by, of a clinical nursing unit which actively pursues research, is available for realistic and clinically based research training, and continuously disseminates knowledge of research findings and implications. This is not to suggest that clinical research be confined to the CNU, but rather that clinical research can be promoted, developed and supported in all of the nursing settings in a district as a result of the unit's activities. Clinical nurses in the hospital and community services may, themselves, begin to utilise research findings, and conduct their own research if the required knowledge and support resources are seen to be readily available and accessible.

The CNU's research activities may be guided by the ideas inherent in the 'centres for clinical nursing research' which Abdellah and Levine (1965) suggest should be established in the USA. They see these centres as units within a larger clinical medical research facility, or as units within a hospital. The purpose of establishing such centres is said to be to provide a research and teaching unit in which the effects of nursing practice can be investigated, and methodologies of nursing practice can be developed. The problems being investigated would be nursing problems, and admission to the unit would be limited to those patients who do not ordinarily require intensive medical care or treatment, arrangements being made with medical staff to provide medical care and evaluation of the patients' medical status as needed. Abdellah and Levine (1965) emphasise that a centre would concentrate on independent nursing studies, but that establishing such centres would not be an attempt to devalue other types of clinical research in which medicine and nursing collaborate. Indeed, research at the clinical level in areas were nurses work collaboratively must be encouraged, and many nursing investigations demand being carried out with patients who are admitted for medical care. With its main research brief of investigating clinical nursing problems, the unit's main teaching brief is to motivate and equip nurses practising in the collaborative nursing settings to carry out research.

Research within the CNU may utilise a variety of methodologies and designs to evaluate nursing quantitatively and qualitatively. The consultant in clinical nursing will be a nurse with preparation in research methods, who is in daily contact with the reality of clinical nursing, and research will be a task of all the unit's staff. Jacox (1974) purports that 'If we are to have knowledge that is useful for practice, then a majority of persons who develop that knowledge must be so familiar with the clinical setting that they are able to identify truly significant problems for study.'

Traditional research methodologies, focusing on objectivity, precision, and adherence to classical designs, may be employed in the unit's programme of research. Less traditional, and newer, methodologies may also have a place, and new methods may be developed and explored. Ketefian (1975) states that 'Few fields appear to have more potential for creative research than nursing', and Bond (1978) asks 'Do we select nursing problems which will fit with accepted "traditional research" methods, or do we develop new methods to fit the particular characteristics of nursing problems?' The methodologies of action research (MacDonald and Otto, 1978) and grounded theory (Glaser and Strauss, 1967) with the researcher as participant, offer valuable insights for the CNU, and the resulting generation of nursing concepts and theories may lead to the construction of new, more applicable methods.

A thorough discussion of the merits and shortcomings of various methodologies is beyond the scope of this book. However, the case for 'triangulation' of research methods put forward by Denzin (1970), who writes from a sociological viewpoint, is useful to the consideration of research in the CNU. 'Triangulation' is the application of different methodologies in a research study to gain maximum data, an approach utilised by Hall (1978). By combining multiple observers' data, and multiple methods, the research effort can to some extent overcome the intrinsic bias in simple-method, simple-observer, simple-theory approaches. Becker's study makes quantitative use of qualitative data, which Denzin (1970) purports 'permits the observer to determine which of his initial propositions are worthy of pursuit'. Such an approach is perhaps the one of choice for a CNU.

The central research concern in the CNU will be that of validating current practices and extending knowledge on how nurses can apply the concepts inherent in the model for nursing on which practice in the unit is based. If, as proposed in Chapter 4, Roper *et al.*'s (1980) model is utilised, the research programme may initially concentrate on the study and exploration of how nurses can best promote self-care for the patient in his activities of living. Abdellah and Levine (1965) suggest there is a great need for research to find out how the concept of self-care can be applied in nursing, and this is an area which may be explored by the CNU. Through its research programme, centred as it is in the heart of practice, the CNU will aim at demonstrating to clinical nurses how, and encourage them to seek knowledge of relationships that will guide action and modify the methods of the very nature of that professional practice.

Still in the realms of research in the CNU, but overlapping with its teaching function, is the dissemination of expertise and knowledge to the whole range of clinical nurses working in the health division or district in which the unit is situated. By concentrating on the production and doing of research, there is a danger that the consumption of research will be neglected, and this would negate the major justification for setting up a CNU. It must be of use to all of the district's nurses, and have some use as an implementor of practice change. Essentially, it serves to effect what Bond (1978) refers to as the 'proletarianisation' of research in nursing. She claims that research studies carried out by 'academic and non-clinically involved nurses has had little impact on practice', and that 'for research to begin to have impact on the practice of nursing, does research activity have to become part of the behaviour of every nurse and not confined to some research elite?' It is proposed here that practising clinical nurses must: be able to interpret and appreciate critically the research findings of others; wish to question practices through research themselves; and must have access to a centre where clinical nurses who are proficient and engaged in research can offer guidance and support, if nursing is to become the 'research based profession' advocated by the Report of the Committee on Nursing (1972). Jacox (1974) observes that 'nursing can never develop a scientific basis for its practice until the practitioners themselves — not just the career researchers — have a great deal more involvement in the research', and Dickoff and James (1968) suggest that until the majority of practising nurses adopt research as part of their conceptual basis for practice, it will have little effect on current nursing norms. Bond (1978) asks 'Should clinicians with research training directly pursue their own research activity or should they spend time in helping others to carry out research? Are there going to be different types of researchers — "real" researchers, those with rigorous preparations, and clinician researchers based in care settings?' If a CNU exists, the 'real' researchers — i.e. the consultants in clinical nursing — will be clinician researchers based in the care setting of the CNU, and the CNU will serve to create an army of more clinician researchers in the wards, departments and community services of the health district. Thus all will be 'real, clinician, researchers'.

71

Treece and Treece (1977) maintain that 'Clinical research absolutely demands involvement for understanding; this suggests that no one is in a more strategic spot to conduct clinical research than the clinical nurse.' They say that clinical nurses have failed to grasp the nettle of clinical research, because of the following reasons.

1. Nurses tend to feel that they are 'too busy' taking care of patients to find time to conduct research.

2. Unless the nurse has had academic training geared toward theoretical conceptions, research may not seem important.

3. Unless the importance of research is learned, nurses may not be able to identify problems that are researchable.

4. Many nurses do not have the academic training necessary to feel confident in carrying out clinical research.

5. The ethics of research frighten some individuals. The requirement to obtain administrative/patient/relative approval for projects may deter some investigators. The fear of harming a patient is an obstacle for other researchers.

6. Unless the administrators of nursing service in health care institutions and agencies are research orientated, the nursing staff tends to feel that it is futile to expect support for nursing research; therefore, nurses have little or no motivation to pursue research.

7. Research takes time, time costs money, and money must be budgeted. That is, research may not be conducted because of a lack of funds.

It is hoped that a CNU may help to overcome some of these existing blocks to clinical nurses pursuing clinical research by: acting as a model; actively providing learning experiences for clinical nurses, nursing students, nurse teachers and nurse managers; guiding clinical nurses in identifying research problems; giving advice and support to clinical nurses in submitting research proposals to permission- and fund-granting bodies; promoting an awareness of the value of utilising research finding; and conducting research. In this process, the CNU will be participating in the development of nursing as an occupation, as, according to Clark and Hockey

(1979), 'Nurses must develop the ability to define their decisions and actions on a scientific rather than intuitive or conventional basis. It is in this ability that their claim to professionalism lies.'

Teaching

The teaching of nurses — students, clinicians, educators and managers — is another major task of the CNU. The generation of interest and understanding of research in the district's clinical nurses has received consideration in the section which precedes this, and forms a large part of the unit's teaching commitment. It is pertinent to repeat Bond's (1978) view on research in nursing to emphasise the need for the CNU to expend a great deal of energy on the teaching of nursing research to clinical nurses: 'I feel that research has made, or is making, very little contribution of practical significance to the improvement of nursing.' She cites the findings of Diers (1972) and Ketefian (1975) to support this view, and nurses with recent experience in direct patient care may well concur. There is a need to convey the practical importance of research to the vast numbers of clinical nurses so that they may begin to regard research as a basis for their practice.

In addition to the research teaching commitment, the unit must also be involved in teaching the practical reality of holistic nursing, and advancement of this through a 'nursing process' approach to care (Marrinner, 1979). The incorporation of these concepts into the practice of nursing is already being strived for by many nurses, particularly educators, and is being promoted by the World Health Organisation. The existence of a unit where these values are held and practised is essential for the change in current attitudes to occur (Ottoway, 1976; Duberley, 1977).

As a basis for change, the CNU may play a crucial role; Donovan (1971) says 'We face the monumental task of raising the sights of the practitioner at every level and in every situation, rural or urban, to a view of intelligent and facile practice of comprehensive nursing care. The great challenge is to get nurses everywhere to assimilate this greatly expanded role and incorporate it into practice. We must raise the base of nursing care above the level of custodial care and the fulfilling of the doctor's orders, to co-ordinated, complete and continuing care.' How, through teaching, can the CNU extend itself into the wider division or district enough to offer the opportunity to clinical nurses to explore nursing itself?

The unit's teaching activities may be directed at two distinct groups: nursing students/pupils and qualified nurses. To consider this more fully, it is necessary to discuss it in the context of teaching basic learners, teaching in the continuing education programmes, the CNU as a teaching unit, and the consultant in clinical nursing as a teacher. The brief of this book is to explore the development of clinical nursing, and thus discussion of educational function of the CNU is essentially brief. However, it must be stressed that education and clinical practice are inextricably entwined in that how nurses practice is greatly influenced by their learning experiences; education for nursing must be based on its practice, and change in practice should create a perception of learning needs in those involved in the change (Ottoway, 1976) — needs which must be met by education if the change is to become a norm in reality.

Basic learners

McFarlane (1977) states that 'Nursing is a practice discipline and the primary objective of education in the profession is education for practice.' In other words, the objective of nursing education is to produce someone who can practise professional nursing. Elhart *et al*. (1978) observe that 'The most significant characteristic of the professional nurse is her ability to make decisions about nursing care.' Infante (1975) depicts professional education as a bridge between the world of thought and that of action, aimed at guiding the student in gaining knowledge of himself, an understanding of the world in which he lives, and knowledge of his area of expertise. The professional practitioner has competence in the practice of the skills related to the services he provides, but these must flow from organised knowledge. Knowledge and an understanding of principles are necessary, according to Bruner (1960), for the practice of all skills. In nursing, nursing knowledge and understanding of nursing principles are prerequisites to the practice of nursing skill (intellectual, psychomotor, or interpersonal) and the provision of a clinical area for practising skills is a prerequisite for mastery (Infante, 1975). Essential for gaining mastery is the practice of skills under competent guidance. In most nursing schools, the clinical area for the practice of skills is traditionally that where patients are nursed, and in the early part of the development of nursing education, caring for patients and the training of nurses were seen as being integral components of the ward or department's activities. More recently, education has withdrawn from service to 'improve' learning experiences for students, and the nurse teacher emerged as a distinct role, the holder of such a post having received preparation in how to transmit knowledge, and gained the knowledge to transmit. There is now an awareness of the fact that nurse teachers are no longer seen to be the persons with expertise in nursing care, and ward sisters express negative views about tutors and their ability to nurse (Duttan, 1978). There now appears to be a great divide between those who *do* the nursing, and those who teach it. Hicks and Westphal (1977) comment that whilst nursing education has now gained a degree of independence, it has, in the process, divorced itself from clinical nursing, despite it being its logical and essential counterpart.

The essential close relationship between theory and practice has lost its closeness, has separated, and is about to be divorced. There thus seems to be a need for reconciliation so that harmony can once again prevail, and meaningful relationships develop. The major aim of the two centres of excellence set up in the USA (Christman, 1980a; Ford, 1980) is to reunite education and service, and in doing so, they are proving that a productive marriage can materialise. Nayer (1980) points out, in describing these centres, that 'Only by having nurses in education and service involved in a three pronged effort — practice, teaching, and research — will nursing care reach its optimum and students acquire attitudes towards care that are truly professional.'

In most situations, however, that a rift exists is undeniable. Davis (1966), in describing the stages of socialisation of student nurses, outlines how a student nurse reconciles herself to the inconsistencies between the teachings of her tutors and the reality of the ward situation.

Many other writers clearly demonstrate this incongruity (e.g. Hunt, 1974; Kramer, 1974; Birch, 1975). The Report of the Committee on Nursing (1972) criticises the tutor who is divorced from the practice of nursing. It is essential to establish some continuity of philosophy between the school and clinical areas, and closer links between service and education need to be formed.

The Royal Commission on the NHS (1979) suggested that the development of 'joint appointments', where teaching and caring functions are combined, may alleviate the gap between education and service. McFarlane (1980b) sees as a most urgent need 'a healing of the breach between education and service to which joint appointments might make a contribution'. Bendall's study, cited by McFarlane, discusses how inadequately nursing education correlates theory and practice and suggests that there is now a need for 'an entirely different approach to the teaching of nursing'. Esther and Bryant (1977) argue for the establishment of joint appointments as a means of raising the quality of patient care, enhancing the learning climate for learners, and fostering the development of research in clinical nursing. Powers (1976), whilst not denying the value of joint appointments, points out major obstacles in establishing them, not least being current strongly held attitudes of tutors and nurse managers.

The role of the consultant in clinical nursing may be seen as a type of joint appointment in that, whilst she is primarily responsible for the nursing of her patients, she has a major clearly defined teaching role. The CNU may be used as an example of the ideal in clinical nursing, operating from the basis of a conceptual model to deliver patient-centred care utilising knowledge gained from nursing research. As such, learner nurses may be allocated to the unit to experience the application of theory in reality, and to have the opportunity for creativity and problem solving in a setting which focuses on nursing. A logical use of these resources would be for the consultant in clinical nursing to teach that component of the basic nurse training courses which covers the elements of nursing theory, and the research component. The very fact that the teacher currently practises what she teaches may lend credibility to her words, and the CNU can be used as a clinical laboratory for the correlation of theory and practice. Beginning learners may practise skills basic to nursing under competent supervision by the consultant in clinical nursing, who introduced them in the classroom. It is feasible to postulate that one of the modules suggested by the Report of the Committee on Nursing (1972), to integrate theoretical and practical teaching, could be designated as an introduction to nursing module, focusing on applying the nursing process based on Roper *et al.*'s (1980) model for nursing. The theoretical input for the module could be provided by the consultant in clinical nursing and unit staff, whilst clinical practice takes place in the CNU. Similarly, when the research component of the basic course is taught by the consultant in clinical nursing, learners may witness the application of research findings to practice and clinical research studies in practice by visiting the CNU. The consultant in clinical nursing may act as a consultant not only to other clinical nurses and health care workers, but also to nurse educators.

Continuing education

Donovan (1971) sees continuing education as a 'powerful force in any project for the uniform mass education of nurses'. Although she acknowledges the usefulness of study days, courses, seminars and literature etc., she sees the best resource as being a 'number of nurses who are prepared and committed to total nursing care to help educate and serve as role models for others'. It is precisely these three activities — helping, educating, and acting as role models — which comprise the input of the consultant in clinical nursing and the

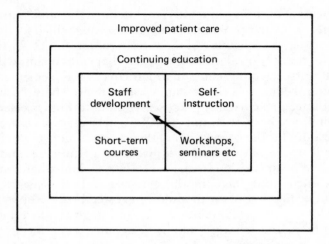

Fig. 8 The relationship of staff development within service and education (from Tobin, 1974).

unit staff in the continuing education programmes of the health district.

The need for continuing education in nursing, particularly to support a change effort, staff development, and the raising of standards, has been well documented (e.g. Cuming, 1975). Tobin (1974) presents a concise and complete analysis of continuing education in nursing, defining it as 'Systematic learning experiences, designed to build upon and to preserve knowledge and skills.' It is said to have two main aspects — in-service education, and staff development — which stem from 'organised planned programmes' and 'individual endeavour'. Figure 8 shows the relationships of these, and how they all serve to improve patient care.

Most health facilities have in-service education officers in post, or a post-basic education unit which provides a continuing education programme. The CNU should develop close links with these educators, and the consultant in clinical nursing should be regarded as a potential member of the in-service education team when programmes are developed. As with her association with the basic nurse training programme, the consultant in clinical nursing and the CNU may serve to offer learning experiences in comprehensive nursing care and nursing research by direct teaching, offering easy access for clinical nurses to work in the unit to meet their perceived learning needs, and by acting as role models for clinical nurses.

Much of the previous discussion on basic nursing education is directly applicable to continuing education. The fact that the consultant in clinical nursing is a practising clinical nurse who does the same, in real terms, as other clinical nurses is likely, again, to give credibility to her teaching. The personal abilities of the consultant in clinical nursing to relate to colleagues in other clinical settings must be such that she does not become alienated from them because of the differences in roles (Ottoway, 1976).

The clinical nursing unit as a teaching unit

The major educational impact to be derived from the unit will be its very presence in the health division or district, as a model nursing unit. The ideals it must project are the importance of clinical nursing research and creative patient care, and the fact that they can be practically applied. Research teaching has already been discussed. The representation of a creative environment conducive to comprehensive nursing care through the utilisation of a problem-solving approach is a requirement of the CNU as an area in which learning can take place.

The unit must provide a means of access to a creative, innovative environment for students and clinicians. It must offer teaching, opportunities for practice, and follow-up support for those who seek it. As such, the CNU should closely identify with both nursing service and nursing education departments. As well as being a building housing patients, staff and equipment, it should also be seen to house a creative environment for clinical nursing.

Schweer (1972) purports that 'If we truly seek to keep creativity alive, we must continue to nourish the conditions in which creativity flourishes.' The CNU must provide these conditions for its own staff, and for nurses elsewhere who choose to utilise them. Schweer (1972) describes four aspects of the creative process, and these four should be promoted and become the norms in the daily working of the CNU, be adopted by the consultant in clinical nursing and, eventually, all unit staff. Schweer proclaims the need to infiltrate the environment, with an emphasis on openness (to new ideas); focus (on direction); discipline (of self to be creative); and closure (when the creative product has been produced).

The practice of nursing within an environment which acknowledges and promotes the four aspects of creativity is the greatest offer of the CNU as a teaching unit to the district it serves.

The consultant in clinical nursing as a teacher

Much of the responsibility in the creation of an environment conducive to learning lies with the consultant in clinical nursing. It is apparent that her role is many faceted, and that she will require extensive experience and preparation to fulfil it. The main requirements for her teaching role are enthusiasm for the development of clinical nursing and a desire to convey this enthusiasm to others. Schweer (1972) succinctly describes what the teacher of clinical nursing should be and do, and this description may sum up the teaching role of the consultant in clinical nursing.

The consultant in clinical nursing as a teacher of creative clinical nursing, is one who does the following.

1. 'Possesses a conceptual model to guide her own thinking and actions.

2. 'Utilises her full potential through a positive, realistic understanding and acceptance of self.

3. 'Possesses a sensitivity and responsiveness to people, ideas and events.

4. 'Exhibits an inner security in dealing with those high-risk situations evolving from the inevitable daily changes and adjustments.

5. 'Recognises the need for continued learning as a necessary ingredient for developing and perfecting her own creative approaches to teaching when challenges arise and new frontiers of learning appear.'

Such a description of the consultant in clinical nursing is perhaps applicable to all of the functions which she is expected to fulfil, and in all of her actions — clinical practice and research included — the consultant in clinical nursing may be seen to be teaching.

7 | Quality Assurance

> Measuring the quality of nursing care is as complex as measuring the quality of professional practice in any field but it is an essential tool of accountability and control.
>
> (Jean McFarlane, *Quality of Nursing Care*)

The CNU aims at providing high quality nursing to those who require it. As such, it is therefore vital to build into its operations a continuous effort to monitor the quality of nursing, and to develop a strategy by which quality of nursing can be controlled, and thus assured.

The terms 'quality assurance' and 'quality control' are increasingly becoming part of the current nursing vocabulary. 'Quality' is defined by the *Kings English Dictionary* (1930) as 'nature or character of, in relation to right or wrong, as of an action; power of effects'. 'Assurance' is said to denote 'freedom from doubt' and 'control' is described as 'to regulate, to govern or direct'. Quality assurance may therefore be interpreted as promising, or making certain of, a standard of excellence. Control is the means by which quality can be assured. Mayers *et al.* (1977) observe that quality assurance has the goal of making certain that nursing practices will produce good patient outcomes. The purpose of quality assurance is, according to Schmadl (1979), to assure the consumer of nursing of a specified degree of excellence through continuous measurement and evaluation.

A number of valid reasons to justify the institution of a quality assurance programme in any nursing context are presented in the literature. The most important, and perhaps obvious, reason must be to promote the provision of a level of nursing which is the right of each individual who seeks, is directed to, or needs the services of a nurse, and therefore provide a means in which accountability for her actions can be approached by the nurse (Egleston, 1980). The need for such measures is increasing, with the growing knowledge of health care consumers and the consequent threat of legal action by individuals or pressure groups — particularly evident in North America. Official bodies responsible for accrediting health care institutions in the USA insist on some form of quality assurance, largely for these very reasons (Egleston, 1980). In addition to the accountability aspect of quality assurance, the development of tools to measure the quality of nursing may very well lead to the development of nursing itself, as they demand a definition of what constitutes nursing, and thus agreement on what is the unique role of the nurse.

Determining the degree of quality of nursing desired, and ensuring that it is achieved, is an important part of the work of the clinical nursing unit, and appraisal of quality is a means of instituting necessary change in the unit aimed at improvement both in the unit and in the wider health division or district. The whole process must be a continuous one of implementation of change and re-evaluation.

Hall (1966) points out that 'prior to any discussion of the quality of nursing care, one must determine what it is that is being evalued. What is nursing?' She goes on to ask 'What methods can we use to evaluate the quality of nursing care? Can we do this by examining the product, i.e. the patient on discharge? Too often we know that the patient recovers in spite of the care he experiences. Can we find out the quality by asking the patient his opinion of it? He may be able to tell us his reactions to the kind he has experienced but unless he has experienced and understood each kind, he will be in no position to help us evaluate. It seems that the most valid method lies in the observation of the process itself.' Hegyvary and Haussman (1976) concur with this view, purporting that the most valid measurement of the quality of nursing is that which focuses on the actual nursing performed in the delivery of care to a patient. The above statement by Hall, however, lays open the field for extensive discussion on how best to measure quality; a topic which is widely discussed and argued about in all of the existing fields of nursing. In considering quality assurance in the CNU, the main methods devised up to the present day are to be reviewed; the various supporting and opposing arguments briefly mentioned; and suggestions made on what methods and instruments may be of use in the CNU.

In addition to the 'process' approach previously mentioned, McFarlane (1980) identifies two other approaches currently in use — the structural evaluation approach, and the outcome-evaluation approach through the use of problem-orientated records. Jelinek *et al*. (1974) describe the structural approach as one which focuses on the physical facilities, organisation and manpower resources of the unit, whilst the outcome approach is said to focus on the patient's welfare and the eventual outcome of care including recovery, mortality rates, and the level of patient satisfaction. Bloch (1975), Mayers *et al*. (1977), and Doughty and Mash (1977) all suggest a combination of the process-evaluation and the outcome-evaluation approaches to constitute a process–outcome approach. This combination may describe the extent to which the achievement of objectives is due to the nursing given.

In all approaches, Berg (1974) suggests that three basic steps must be ascended in the overall programme:

define what should be present
compare what should be with what is
identify the gaps and take action.

Defining what should be present is perhaps the most difficult step, and may well be a subject of much contention and disagreement. It is considered, somewhat briefly, later in this chapter when specific instruments are described. Comparing what should be with what is requires a method of collecting data to establish what is. Two methods of data collection are identified in the literature — retrospective and concurrent. The former utilises a review of the nursing given after it is completed, whereas the latter occurs whilst the nursing is still in progress. Retrospective evaluation of the quality of nursing may be effected by (Mayers *et al*., 1977):

post-care patient interview
post-care patient questionnaire
post-care staff conference
audit of the records.

84

Concurrent evaluation may be effected by:

assessment of the outcomes of care
patient interviews
conference between patient, staff and relatives
direct observation of care
measurement of the competency of the nurse
audit of the records.

Much has been written on the 'best' method of quality care evaluation, and various writers argue in favour of a specific approach whilst validly criticising methods which do not meet their approval. It is reasonable to suggest that an effective quality assurance programme may need to use several methods, and that, indeed, to do so may increase effectiveness (Hover and Zimmer, 1978). Methods encompassing a process and outcome approach may be those of choice for a clinical nursing unit, exploring, as they do, the nursing activity within the unit and its effect on the ultimate outcomes (Bloch, 1975). Tools utilising retrospective and concurrent methods, and focusing on both process and outcome, are suggested, and three tools which, if used together, will do this are to be described.

Outcome approach

Mayers *et al.* (1977) describe how quality of care can be measured according to whether or not stated outcomes of care are set. Other authors prefer to use the term objectives, and McFarlane (1980) suggests that the use of problem-orientated records facilitates evaluation by the outcome approach. This method may be used concurrently or retrospectively. It is often used concurrently as part of the nursing process, and Mayers *et al.* (1977) see it as part of the evaluation component of the nursing process. To be effective, it is essential that the outcome desired is stated in specific behavioural terms and that the observable behaviour stated should be measurable. Mager (1962) outlines how behavioural objectives should be stated, within the context of

Table 6   Example of an item on a nursing care plan

Problem	Plan	Expected outcome	Target date
Unable to give own daily dose of insulin	1. Daily teaching programme/ demonstration on technique at 4 p.m. 2. Allow patient 'space' to discuss his fears about the procedure and to explore his own feelings 3. Offer him the opportunity to give own injections each day, without applying pressure	Will give correct dose of insulin, using correct, technique. Express a wish to do this permanently	12.12.82

education, but directly applicable to nursing care plans, and applying his basic requisites of objectives to the statement of patient outcomes is of value in setting criteria as a measure of quality nursing. The statement should state:

what the patient will do
at what level of proficiency
and under what circumstances.

Mayers *et al.* (1977) suggest that a target date or deadline for achievement of the objective or outcome should be written. As an example, an item on the nursing care plan may be as shown in Table 6.

When nursing care plans are written in this way, it is relatively easy to evaluate the care given in terms of whether or not the expected outcomes are achieved, on or before the target date. This may be undertaken for all patients at regular intervals, or for randomly selected patients regularly or sporadically. Retrospectively, all or selected care plans can be evaluated on the basis of outcomes, for discharged patients.

Quality of patient care scale

The quality of patient care scale, or Qualpacs (Wandelt and Ager, 1974), concentrates on the process of nursing by considering the nursing given by direct observation. It is suggested by many that this is the only valid way to assess quality of nursing care. Wandelt and Ager (1974) claim that Qualpacs is an instrument which can measure the quality of care received by a patient in any setting. It consists of 68 items, in chart form, arranged into six subsections.

1. *Psychosocial: individual* (15 items). 'Actions directed toward meeting psychosocial needs of individual patients.'

2. *Psychosocial: group* (8 items). 'Actions directed toward meeting psychosocial needs of patients as members of a group.'

3. *Physical* (15 items). 'Actions directed toward meeting the physical needs of patients.'

4. *General* (15 items). 'Actions directed toward meeting either psychosocial or physical needs of the patient, or both at the same time.'

5. *Communication* (8 items). 'Communication on behalf of the patient.'

6. *Professional implications* (7 items). 'Care given to patients reflects initiative and responsibility indicative of professional expectations.'

Each individual item is accompanied by a concise statement of an action, and a 20-page 'cue sheet' gives specific examples of such activities to assist the rater. A full explanatory text outlines the whole procedure for raters and implementors of the Qualpacs scale. Two or more observer raters are suggested for an observation of care in any setting for a period of two hours, and to evaluate care by all who give it, and not only one care giver. Thus, Qualpacs attempts to measure total care given during the observation period.

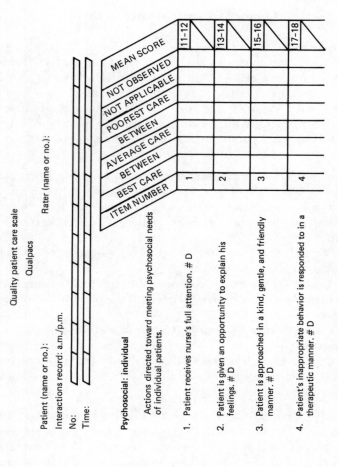

Quality patient care scale

Qualpacs

Patient (name or no.):

Rater (name or no.):

Interactions record: a.m./p.m.

No:

Time:

Psychosocial: individual

Actions directed toward meeting psychosocial needs of individual patients.

ITEM NUMBER	BEST CARE	BETWEEN	AVERAGE CARE	BETWEEN	POOREST CARE	NOT APPLICABLE	NOT OBSERVED	MEAN SCORE
1								11-12
2								13-14
3								15-16
4								17-18

1. Patient receives nurse's full attention. # D

2. Patient is given an opportunity to explain his feelings. # D

3. Patient is approached in a kind, gentle, and friendly manner. # D

4. Patient's inappropriate behavior is responded to in a therapeutic manner. # D

Fig. 9   Example of the Qualpacs scale.

Basically, Wandelt and Ager (1974) state that the raters must familiarise themselves with the rating scale by using it for approximately two days, having previously read the text, and by using the two days to gain observational skill, discuss questions on acceptable standards, and establish shared concepts of these standards. They suggest that assessment of care should be carried out on selected patients, using a random numbers' table for selecting from those who are expected to be involved in a number of nurse–patient interactions during the observation period. Immediately before the observation, the raters establish a knowledge base about the patient concerned by communicating with nursing staff, reviewing the patient's records, and by developing an assessment base and care plan. The raters are then introduced to the patient by the nurse, the procedure explained, and consent obtained. Throughout the observation, the raters record their judgements on the Qualpacs scale. As an example, part of the scale is shown in Fig. 9.

All interactions with the patient are recorded, and may include various staff members of different levels. Similarly, several recordings may be made in a single rating space. At the end of the observation, a mean score is arrived at from the total number of items relevant to the observation, and the numerical Qualpacs score can be equated to a descriptive statement:

1 = poorest care
2 = between
3 = average care
4 = between
5 = best care.

The Qualpacs scale attempts to evaluate the process of care as it occurs in reality— by direct observation— and offers an opportunity to benefit the receivers of care whilst it is still in progress. Many writers purport that direct observation of care is the only realistic way to affect the care of patients who are currently being nursed, and that this aspect of quality assurance is one of importance. As a tool, Qualpacs has been extensively tested for reliability and validity and appears to offer a valuable framework for part of a quality assurance programme in settings where a holistic approach to nursing is part of the current philosophy.

Nursing audit

Phaneuf (1976) describes the nursing audit as being a process-orientated approach to appraise the nursing process as it is reflected in the patients' records, and as a retrospective method of quality assurance. The audit plan, to be used by the auditors, utilises the functions of nursing listed by Lesnik and Anderson (1955).

1. The application and execution of the doctor's legal orders.
2. The observation of symptoms and reactions.
3. Supervision of the patients.
4. Supervision of those participating in care.
5. Reporting and recording.
6. The application of nursing procedures and techniques.
7. The promotion of health by directing and teaching.

From these seven functions, Phaneuf (1976) identifies 50 components to help auditors evaluate the quality of nursing by 'focusing their attention on the patient rather than on the nursing specialities or the nurses who administer care' (Marrinner, 1979). The 50 components are stated in terms of actions by nurses in relation to the patient, and in the form of questions to be answered by the auditors as they review the patient's record.

In implementing audit as a method of quality assurance, the setting up of a nursing audit committee is recommended to serve as the 'professional nursing conscience of the agency concerned through its monthly performance of audits'. The committee should have at least five members, and each member should possess clinical competence, commitment to clinical nursing, an interest in quality control, and an ability to work in a group. It is suggested that each member should review no more than ten patients each month, and that an

Part I. HOSPITAL OR NURSING HOME AUDIT

Data must be held in STRICT confidence and MUST NOT BE FILED with patient's record

All Entries To Be Completed By Trained Clerk

1. Name of patient: 2. Sex   3. Age   4. Date admitted   5. Discharge date

   (LAST)   (FIRST)

6. Name of institution: 7. Floor   8.   Medical   Private   Ward   OPD/Clinic
                                          supervision   ☐   ☐   ☐

9. Complete diagnosis(es):

10. Admitted by   Physician   M.D. not hospital   Clinic/OPD   11. Via emergency
    referral from: on staff   affiliated
                     ☐   ☐   ☐   ☐

12. Patient discharged to: Self-care   Family care   PHN Agency   Other   Died   Unknown
                             ☐   ☐   ☐   specify: ☐   ☐
                                                                    ☐

13. If patient died: M.D.   M.D. promptly   Family   Family promptly   14. If patient
                       present   notified   present   notified   Catholic:
                       ☐   ☐   ☐   ☐   Last rites   YES   NO
                                                                                 given: ☐   ☐

15. All nursing entries signed   YES   NO   16.   Nursing entries show whether   YES   NO
    by name and dated: made by professional, practi- ☐   ☐
                                 ☐   ☐   cal, student nurse, or other:

17. Patient's clothing, valuables, and other personal   YES   NO
    items were accounted for in accordance with policy: ☐   ☐

		YES	NO
18.	Operative and other patient or family consent forms completed as required by policy	—	—
19.	A. Were there any accidents or other special incidents?	—	—
	B. If yes, chart indicates report was submitted to administration	—	—
	C. Or, report is part of chart	—	—
20.	A. Kardex in use	—	—
	B. If yes, Kardex becomes part of permanent chart	—	—
21.	Nursing care plan is recorded in the chart	—	—
22.	A. Nursing admission entry shows assessment of patient's condition: physical	—	—
	emotional	—	—
	B. Nursing discharge entry shows assessment of patient's condition: physical	—	—
	emotional	—	—

Fig. 10 Phaneuf's (1976) audit, part 1 (hospital).

PART I. PUBLIC HEALTH NURSING AUDIT

Data must be held in STRICT confidence and MUST NOT BE FILED with patient's record

All Entries To Be Completed by Trained Clerk

1. Name of patient:

   (LAST)   (FIRST)

   2. Sex   3. Age   4. Admission date   5. Discharge date

6. Nursing agency: 7. Number of visits to patient by agency:

8. Complete diagnosis(es):

9. Was patient hospitalized immediately prior to PHN service:
   YES No. days NO Unknown
   ☐   ☐   ☐   ☐

   10. Medical supervision:
   Private Ward OPD/Clinic
   ☐   ☐   ☐

11. Patient referred to PHN by:
    Hospital Hospital
    Nurse Social Worker M.D. Patient's Family Other, specify: Unknown
    ☐   ☐   ☐   ☐   ☐   ☐

12. Patient discharged from PHN to:
    Family
    Self-care care Rehospitalized Died Other PHN agency Other, specify: Unknown
    ☐   ☐   ☐   ☐   ☐   ☐   ☐

13. All nursing entries signed by name and dated:
    YES NO
    ☐   ☐

    14. Nursing entries show whether made by public health, professional, practical, student nurse, physiotherapist, other: YES NO
    ☐   ☐

15. Nursing care plan is recorded: YES NO
    ☐   ☐

		YES	NO
16. Were there any accidents or special incidents?		—	—
A. If yes, chart indicates report was submitted to administration		—	—
B. Or, report is part of the chart		—	—
17. Nursing admission entry shows assessment of patient's condition:	physical	—	—
	emotional	—	—
18. Nursing discharge entry shows assessment of patient's condition:	physical	—	—
	emotional	—	—

Fig. 11 Phaneuf's (1976) audit, part 1 (community).

PART II. NURSING AUDIT CHART REVIEW SCHEDULE

All Entries To Be Completed By A Member Of the Nursing Audit Committee
(Please check in box of choice; DO NOT obscure number in box.)

Name of Patient: _____
(LAST)   (FIRST)

	YES	NO	UNCERTAIN	TOTALS
I. APPLICATION AND EXECUTION OF PHYSICIAN'S LEGAL ORDERS				
1. Medical diagnosis complete	7	0	3	
2. Orders complete	7	0	3	
3. Orders current	7	0	3	
4. Orders promptly executed	7	0	3	
5. Evidence that nurse understood cause and effect	7	0	3	
6. Evidence that nurse took health history into account	7	0	3	
(42) TOTALS		0		☐
II. OBSERVATION OF SYMPTOMS AND REACTIONS				
7. Related to course of above disease(s) in general	7	0	3	
8. Related to course of above disease(s) in patient	7	0	3	
9. Related to complications due to therapy (each medication and each procedure)	7	0	3	
10. Vital signs	7	0	3	
11. Patient to his condition	7	0	3	
12. Patient to his course of disease(s)	5	0	2	
(40) TOTALS		0		☐
III. SUPERVISION OF THE PATIENT				
13. Evidence that initial nursing diagnosis was made	4	0	1	
14. Safety of patient	4	0	1	
15. Security of patient	4	0	1	
16. Adaptation (support of patient in reaction to condition and care)	4	0	1	
17. Continuing assessment of patient's condition and capacity	4	0	1	
18. Nursing plans changed in accordance with assessment	4	0	1	
19. Interaction with family and with others considered	4	0	1	
(28) TOTALS		0		☐
IV. SUPERVISION OF THOSE PARTICIPATING IN CARE (EXCEPT THE PHYSICIAN)				
20. Care taught to patient, family, or others, nursing personnel	5	0	2	
21. Physical, emotional, mental capacity to learn considered	5	0	2	
22. Continuity of supervision to those taught	5	0	2	
23. Support of those giving care	5	0	2	
(20) TOTALS		0		☐
V. REPORTING AND RECORDING				
24. Facts on which further care depended were recorded	4	0	1	
25. Essential facts reported to physician	4	0	1	
26. Reporting of facts included evaluation thereof	4	0	1	
27. Patient or family alerted as to what to report to physician	4	0	1	
28. Record permitted continuity of intramural and extramural care	4	0	1	
(20) TOTALS		0		☐

Fig. 12 Phaneuf's (1976) audit, part 2.

VI. APPLICATION AND EXECUTION OF NURSING PROCEDURES AND TECHNIQUES

	YES	NO	UNCERTAIN	TOTALS	DOES NOT APPLY
29. Administration and/or supervision of medications	2	0	0.5		2
30. Personal care (bathing, oral hygiene, skin, nail care, shampoo)	2	0	0.5		2
31. Nutrition (including special diets)	2	0	0.5		2
32. Fluid balance plus electrolytes	2	0	0.5		2
33. Elimination	2	0	0.5		2
34. Rest and sleep	2	0	0.5		2
35. Physical activity	2	0	0.5		2
36. Irrigations (including enemas)	2	0	0.5		2
37. Dressings and bandages	2	0	0.5		2
38. Formal exercise program	2	0	0.5		2
39. Rehabilitation (other than formal exercise)	2	0	0.5		2
40. Prevention of complications and infections	2	0	0.5		2
41. Recreation, diversion	2	0	0.5		2
42. Clinical procedures — urinalysis, B/P	2	0	0.5		2
43. Special treatments (e.g., care of tracheotomy, use of oxygen, colostomy or catheter care, etc.)	2	0	0.5		2
44. Procedures and techniques taught to patient	2	0	0.5		2
(32) TOTALS		0		☐	

VII. PROMOTION OF PHYSICAL AND EMOTIONAL HEALTH BY DIRECTION AND TEACHING

	YES	NO	UNCERTAIN	TOTALS	DOES NOT APPLY
45. Plans for medical emergency evident	3	0	1		3
46. Emotional support to patient	3	0	1		3
47. Emotional support to family	3	0	1		3
48. Teaching promotion and maintenance of health	3	0	1		3
49. Evaluation of need for additional resources (e.g., spiritual, social service, homemaker service, physical or occupational therapy)	3	0	1		3
50. Action taken in regard to needs identified	3	0	1		3
(18) TOTALS		0		☐	

TOTAL SCORE ☐

FINAL SCORE ☐

auditor will be able to carry out a single audit in approximately 15 minutes when skill in using the method is acquired. If the number of discharges per month is less than 50, all may be audited, but when larger numbers are involved, patients may be selected so that 10% of discharges are reviewed.

The instrument constructed for the use of auditors to evaluate systematically the care given as recorded in the records comprises three parts. Part one refers to the setting, and two separate formats are presented by Phaneuf — one specifically for hospital or nursing home care, and the other for community-based care (Figs. 10 and 11).

Phaneuf recommends that this section be completed by a member of the clerical staff as its completion does not demand nursing judgement. The items in it are not scored, although they may be referred to in the later parts of the audit.

Part two is the chart review schedule, and comprises the 50 components derived from the seven nursing functions outlined previously and posed in terms of questions to be answered by the auditors. In answering each question, provision is made for the auditor to respond with 'uncertain' and, in some items, 'does not apply' (Fig. 12). The audit committee decides on what criteria they will accept as having met the requirements of each component. After completion of part two, the reply on each question is scored, and the score is then weighted according to the relative importance assigned to the component concerned. Phaneuf maintains that the weighting system has been derived from extensive testing of the instrument.

The final audit score is arrived at by multiplying the total score of individual component scores by a value determined by the 'does not apply' responses, and is entered on part three of the audit document. The final, numerical audit score is equated with one of five descriptive statements:

161–200 = excellent
121–160 = good
  81–120 = incomplete
  41–80 = poor
   0–40 = unsafe.

95

The nursing audit of patient records has been widely criticised as a method of quality assurance. Hegyvary and Haussman (1976) purport that it only serves to improve documentation, not nursing care, and Mayers *et al.*(1977) see its major fault as being its assumption that what is done is documented, and what is documented is done. Phaneuf (1976) suggests that good documentation leads to good nursing, but Jelineck *et al.*(1974) argue that nurses soon learn how to document in a way which favourably influences the audit results, without necessarily changing the delivery of nursing. Despite the arguments, nursing audit may be useful as part of, but not necessarily as the total means of, a quality assurance programme if the records in use are accurate records of care. Records in current use in most British nursing situations are not likely to be suitable (Lelean, 1973). In units, like the proposed CNU, where nursing records follow a nursing process approach, nursing audit may be a feasible and desirable component of an effort to evaluate the quality of nursing.

The various approaches to quality assurance described in the literature all appear to offer some specific direction when an attempt to promise a degree of excellence in nursing care is desired, but it is reasonable to assume that the use of a single method may not be the total answer (Zimmer, 1980). Nevertheless, many of the tools devised set out a specific and systematic way to promote the maintenance and raising of standards of care, albeit each concentrates on a different aspect (Block, 1975; McClure, 1976; Doughty and Mash, 1977; Moore, 1979). An amalgam of approaches is seen as the most useful strategy in the CNU until more satisfactory, all-embracing methods emerge— if such an event does occur.

It is suggested here that the patient outcome approach utilising problem-orientated records, the quality patient care scale, and the nursing audit, all be used in a quality assurance programme in the CNU.

The use of such a combination will allow for the nursing process, and the outcomes of this, to be evaluated, both concurrently and retrospectively, in the drive with which nurses have traditionally identified — to improve and maintain the quality of the care they provide (Egleston, 1980) — and which is the fundamental purpose of a CNU.

8 | Conclusion

There warn't anybody at the church, except maybe a hog or two, for there warn't any lock on the door, and hogs like a puncheon floor in summertime because it's cool. If you notice, most folks don't go to church, only when they've got to; but a hog is different.
(Mark Twain, *Adventures of Huckleberry Finn*)

The shrewd guess, the fertile hypothesis, the courageous leap to a tentative conclusion — these are the most valuable coin of the thinker at work.
(Jerome Seymore Bruner, *The Process of Education*)

Clinical nurses today, with support from nurse managers, educators, and researchers, are seeking to strengthen their role and to establish a career structure for clinical nurses, and expansive discussion is currently taking place on how such a structure can be constructed. Individual nurses and health care facilities are implementing innovative strategies both to promote the recognition of clinical nursing and to create roles which expand the role of the nurse and unify practice, research and teaching.

Developing a structure and work environment to accommodate advanced clinical roles is a task of immense complexity. This book is an attempt to outline one framework which would allow clinical nurses who have acquired experience and a broad educational background the choice to progress to positions affording greater autonomy and financial reward, whilst remaining in direct contact with those who need nursing. An attempt to implement this framework is currently in progress at Burford Community Hospital and Nursing Development Unit in Oxfordshire.

The clinical nurse specialist role is supported, and it is suggested that this role should be promoted. The major concern, however, has been the development of a higher level role of a consultant in clinical nursing, based in a clinical nursing unit. In order to present a total representation of the concept of the CNU, nursing within it has been discussed, focusing on its practice, work organisation, research, teaching, and effort to ensure quality of care.

The purpose of this book is to stimulate discussion on the development of clinical nursing, and not to provide an answer to nursing's most difficult contemporary task. Indeed, the open mind is perhaps the greatest asset to today's planners and leaders. Postulating narrow, unchangeable views does not promote change, but the presentation of ideas accompanied by the ability to question and reform them is the only way in which creative development in nursing can evolve. If this book were to be rewritten, much would probably need to be altered, as the writer's views change as a result of the continuing work at Burford.

If clinical nursing is to develop in order to provide the quality of nursing which is the right of all individuals, the vast number of nurses who practise today must be motivated to think and talk about nursing as a discipline; to consider the implications of individualised, holistic care; and to develop advanced clinical roles creatively.

Nursing is the direct interaction between helper and helped, and when those who are engaged in this are afforded the same status as their colleagues who manage resources and educate nurses, the practice of nursing will be recognised as the central concern for those who are known as nurses.

References

Abdellah F., Beland I.L., Martin A., Matheney R.V. (1960). *Patient Centred Approaches to Nursing*. New York: Macmillan.

Abdellah F.G., Levine E. (1965). *Better Patient Care through Nursing Research*. New York: Macmillan.

Academy of Nursing Meets: Nurses urged to Join with Consumers (1975). *American Nurse;* **8** (10):1.

Alfano G.J. (1969). A professional approach to nursing practice. *Nursing Clinics of North America;* **4**(3):487.

Alfano G.J. (1971). Healing or caretaking — which will it be? *Nursing Clinics of North America;* **6**:273.

Anderson E. (1973). *The Role of the Nurse*. London: Royal College of Nursing.

Ashley J.A. (1975). Nurses in American history. Nursing and early feminism. *American Journal of Nursing*; **75**:149.

Ashworth P. (1975). An English viewpoint — paper presented at Leeds Castle Seminar. In *New Horizons in Clinical Nursing* pp. 11–14. London: Royal College of Nursing.

Bailey J.T., Clauss J.E. (1975). *Decision Making in Nursing*. St Louis, Miss: C.V. Mosby.

Barrett J. (1968). *The Head Nurse — Her Changing Role*, 2nd edn. New York: Appleton-Century-Crofts.

Batchelor I. (1980). *The Multi-disciplinary Clinical Team — a Working Paper*. London: Kings Fund.

Beland I.L. (1970). *Clinical Nursing: Pathophysiological and Psychosocial Approaches*. London: Collier Macmillan.

Berg H. (1974). Evaluation of nursing care in terms of process and outcome. *Journal of Nursing Administration;* **9**:2.

Beyers M., Phillips C. (1971). *Nursing Management for Patient Care*. Boston: Little, Brown.

Bhola H.S. (1975). The design of (educational) policy: directing and harnessing social power for social outcomes. *Viewpoints;* **51**(3):2.

Birch J. (1975). *To Nurse or not to Nurse*. London: Royal College of Nursing.

Blake M. (1980). The Peplau developmental model for nursing practice. In *Conceptual Models for Nursing Practice* (Riehl J.P., Roy C., eds.) pp. 53–59. New York: Appleton-Century-Crofts.

Bloch D. (1977). Criteria, standards, norms. *Journal of Nursing Administration*; September 1977.

Bond S. (1978). Dilemmas in clinical research. Paper presented at Northern Regional Health Authority Seminar on *Developments in Nursing*. Unpublished.

Brenham R.O.J. (1971). Training for ward management. *Nursing Mirror;* **12**:1.

British Geriatrics Society (1976). *Doctors and Old Age*. London: British Geriatrics Society.

Bruner J. (1960). *The Process of Education*. Harvard, Mass: Harvard University Press.

Burdge L. (1978). The role of the clinical nursing officer. *Nursing Times;* **74**(31):1299.

Calley M.M., Dirssen M., Engalla M., Hennrich M.L. (1980). The Orem self-care nursing model. In *Conceptual Models for Nursing Practice* (Riehl J.P., Roy C., eds.) pp. 302–314. New York: Appleton-Century-Crofts.

Carnevali D. (1973). Conceptualising: storage of knowledge for diagnosis and management. In *Concepts Basic to Nursing*, 3rd edn. (Mitchel P.H., Luustav, A., eds.) pp. 207–219. New York: McGraw Hill.

Carr-Saunders A.M., Wilson P.A. (1933). *The Professions*. London: Frank Cass. (Reprinted 1964.)

Chin R. (1980). The utility of systems models and developmental models for practitioners. In *Conceptual Models for Nursing Practice* (Riehl J.P., Roy C., eds.) pp. 21–37. New York: Appleton-Century-Crofts.

Chrisman M.K., Fowler M.D. (1980). The systems-in-change model for nursing practice. In *Conceptual Models for Nursing Practice* (Riehl J.P., Roy C., eds.) pp. 74-102. New York: Appleton-Century-Crofts.

Christman L. (1978a). Accountability and autonomy are more than rhetoric. *Nurse Education;* **3**(4):3.

Christman L. (1978b). Future developments in nursing. Paper presented at 1978 *Forum on Doctoral Education in Nursing*, 29 June. Illinois: Rush University.

Christman L. (1980a). Problems of role definition in the health care team — nursing role. In *Current Perspectives in Nursing*, Vol. 2 (Miller M.H., Flynn B.C., eds.) pp. 15–19. St Louis, Miss: C.V. Mosby.

Christman L. (1980b). *The Organisational Perspective for Nursing Practice*. Paper presented at ANA Convention, 9–13 June, Houston, Texas. Unpublished.

Clark J.M., Hockey L. (1979). *Research for Nursing*. Aylesbury: HM & M.

Cleary J. (1977). The distribution of nursing attention in a children's ward. *Nursing Times* (Occasional paper); 14 July.

Coleman L.J. (1980). Orem's self-care concept of nursing. In *Conceptual Models for Nursing Practice* (Riehl J.P., Roy C., eds.) pp. 315–28. New York: Appleton-Century-Crofts.

Cox S. (1978). The introduction of nurse specialists. *Nursing Times;* **74**(27):1125.

Cuming M.W. (1975). Personnel management. In *A Guide for Teachers of Nurses* (Raybould E., ed.) pp. 88–105. London: Blackwell.

Davies C. (1976). Experience of dependency and control in work: the case of nurses. *Journal of Advanced Nursing;* **1**(4):273.

Davies C. (1977). Continuities in the development of hospital nursing in Britain. *Journal of Advanced Nursing;* **2**(5):479.

Davis F. (1966). Professional socialisation a subjective experience. In *A Sociology of Medical Practice* (Cox C., Mead A., eds.) pp. 116–130. London: Collier Macmillan.

Denzin N.K. (1970). *The Research Act in Sociology*. London: Butterworths.

Department of Health and Social Security (1980). *Nursing Homes: Their Role in the Care of Elderly People*. London: HMSO.

Dickoff J., James P. (1968). Researching research's role in theory development. *Nursing Research;* **17**:204.

Diers D. (1972). Applications of research to nursing practice. *Image;* **5**(2):7.

Donovan H.J. (1971). Is the delivery system of health care the crucial problem in nursing service? *Journal of Nursing Administration;* March/April.

Doughty D.B., Mash N.J. (1977). *Nursing Audit*. Philadelphia: Davis.

Duberley J. (1977). How will the change strike you and me? *Nursing Times;* **73**(45):1736.

Duttan A. (1978). *Factors Affecting Recruitment of Nurse Tutors*. London: Kings Fund.

Egleston E.M. (1980). New JCHH Standard on quality assurance. *Nursing Research;* **29**:2.

Elhart D., Firsich S.C., Gragg S.H., Rees O.M. (1978). *Scientific Principles in Nursing*, 8th edn. St Louis, Miss: C.V. Mosby.

Elpern E.H. (1977). Structural and organisational supports for primary nursing. *Nursing Clinics of North America;* **12**:2.

Esther A.C., Bryant R.J. (1977). Educating the learner to work on the ward. *Nursing Times;* **73**(2):47.

Etzioni A. (1969). *The Semi-professions and their Organisation.* London: Collier Macmillan.

Ford L.C. (1980). Unification of nursing practice, education and research. *Nursing Review;* **27**:6.

Friedson E. (1975). *The Profession of Medicine.* New York; Dodds, Mead.

Glaser B., Strauss A. (1967). *The Discovery of Grounded Theory.* London: Weidenfeld and Nicholson.

Gonzalez F. (1981). How should nursing be managed below the level of director of nursing services? *Nursing Times;* **77**:14.

Hall D.J. (1978). What nurse don't see, she don't worry about— or the use of observation in hospital research. *Nursing Times;* **74**(49), Occasional paper 34:137.

Hall L.E. (1963). A center for nursing. *Nursing Outlook;* **11**:805.

Hall L.E. (1964). *Project Report. The Soloman and Betty Loeb Center at Montefiore Hospital.* New York: Loeb Center for Nursing.

Hall L.E. (1966). Another view of nursing care and quality. In *Continuity of Patient Care: the Role of Nurses* (Straub M., Parker K., eds.) pp. 47–61. Washington DC: Catholic University of America Press.

Hall L.E. (1969). The Loeb Center for Nursing and Rehabilitation, Montefiore Hospital and Medical Center, Bronx, New York. *International Journal of Nursing Studies;* **6**:81.

Hall L.E., Alfano G.J., Rifkin E., Levine H.S. (1975). *Longitudinal Effects of an Experimental Nursing Process.* New York: Loeb Center for Nursing.

Hamilton-Smith S. (1972). *Nil by Mouth.* London: Royal College of Nursing.

Hardy M.E., ed. (1973). *Theoretical Foundations for Nursing.* New York: MSS Information Corp.

Harrington H.A., Theis E.C. (1968). Institutional factors perceived by baccalaureat graduates as influencing their performance as staff nurses. *Nursing Research;* **17**:229.

Hawthorn P. (1974). *Nurse I Want My Mummy.* London: Royal College of Nursing.

Hayward J. (1975). *Information — a Prescription Against Pain.* London: Royal College of Nursing.

Hegyvary S.T., Haussman R.K.D. (1976). Monitoring nursing care quality. *Journal of Nursing Administration;* **6**:9.

Henderson C. (1964). Can nursing care hasten recovery? *American Journal of Nursing;* **64**(6):77.

Henderson V. (1966). *The Nature of Nursing*. London: Collier Macmillan.

Hicks B.C., Westphal M. (1977). Integration of clinical and academic nursing at the hospital clinical unit level. *Journal of Nurse Education;* **16**(4):6.

HMSO (1971). *Better Services for the Mentally Handicapped*. London: HMSO.

HMSO (1972). *Nurses in an Integrated Health Service*. Edinburgh: HMSO.

Holmlund B.A. (1967). *Nursing Study: Phase One*. Saskatoon: University of Saskatchewan.

Hover J., Zimmer M.J. (1978). Nursing quality assurance: the Wisconsin System. *Nursing Outlook;* **26**:4.

Hunt J. (1974). *The Teaching and Practice of Surgical Dressings in Three Hospitals*. London: Royal College of Nursing.

Infante M.S. (1975). *The Clinical Laboratory in Nurse Education*. New York: Wiley.

Jacox A. (1974). Nursing research and the clinician. *Nursing Outlook;* **22**:82.

Jelinek D., Haussman R., Hegyvary S. (1974). *A Methodology for Monitoring Quality of Nursing Care*. Bethesda: US Department of Health.

Johnson B.E. (1980). The behavioural system model for nursing. In *Conceptual Models for Nursing Practice* (Riehl J.P., Roy C., eds.) pp. 207–216. New York: Appleton-Century-Crofts.

Kerrane T.A. (1975a). Role relations. In *New Horizons in Clinical Nursing* pp. 15–16. London: Royal College of Nursing.

Kerrane T.A. (1975b). The clinical nurse specialist. *Nursing Mirror;* **140**(5):63.

Ketefian S. (1975). Application of selected nursing research findings into nursing practice: a pilot study. *Nursing Research;* **24**:2.

Kings English Dictionary (1930). London: British Book Co.

Kohnke H.M. (1978). *The Case for Consultation in Nursing*. New York: Wiley.

Kramer H. (1974). *Reality Shock*. St Louis. Miss: C.V. Mosby.

Kratz C. (1977). The nursing process. *Nursing Times;* **73**(23):854.

Kron T. (1972). *Communication in Nursing*. Philadelphia: W.B. Saunders.

Kron T. (1976). *The Management of Patient Care*. Philadelphia: W.B. Saunders.

Lambertson E.C. (1953). *Nursing Team Organisation and Functioning*. New York: Columbia University Press.

Leino A. (1951). Organising the nursing team. *American Journal of Nursing;* **51**:665.

Lelean S. (1973). *Ready for Report Nurse*. London: Royal College of Nursing.

Leone L.P. (1962). *A New Dedication of Creative Nursing*. Address given at opening of Loeb Center for Nursing, New York, 29 November. Unpublished.

Lesnik M.J., Anderson B.E. (1955). *Nursing Practice and the Laboratory*. Philadelphia: Lippincott.

McClure M.L. (1976). Quality assurance and nursing education. *Nursing Outlook;* **24**:6.

MacDonald I., Otto S. (1978). A way to ensure research is meaningful to the practitioner. *Health and Social Services Journal;* **88**:366.

McFarlane J.K. (1976). The role of research and the development of nursing theory. *Journal of Advanced Nursing;* **1**:443.

McFarlane J.K. (1977). Developing a theory of nursing: the relation of theory to practice, education and research. *Journal of Advanced Nursing;* **2**:261.

McFarlane J. (1980a). *The Multi-disciplinary Team*. London: Kings Fund.

McFarlane J. (1980b). *Essays on Nursing*. London: Kings Fund.

MacGuire J.M. (1980). *The Expanded Role of the Nurse*. London: Kings Fund.

Mager R.F. (1962). *Preparing Instructional Objectives*. Belmont, California: Fearon.

Manthey M. (1970). The history and development of primary nursing. *Nursing Forum;* **IX**(4):359.

Manthey M. (1973). Primary nursing is alive and well in the hospital. *American Journal of Nursing;* **727**(1):83.

Manthey M., Ciske K., Robertson P. (1970). Primary nursing. *Nursing Forum;* **IX**(1):65.

Marram G. (1979). Perspectives in nursing management. In *Primary Nursing*, vol. 1 (Marrinner A., ed.) pp. 84–92. St Louis, Miss: C.V. Mosby.

Marrinner A. (1979). *The Nursing Process*, 2nd edn. St Louis, Miss: C.V. Mosby.

Mayers M.G. (1972). *A Systematic Approach to the Nursing Care Plan*. New York: Appleton-Century-Crofts.

Menzies I.E.P. (1960). Nurses under stress: a social system functioning as a defence against anxiety. *International Nursing Review;* **1**(6):9.

Moore K.R. (1979). What nurses learn from nursing audit. *Nursing Outlook;* **27**(4):254.

Nayer D.D. (1980). Unification. *American Journal of Nursing;* **80**(6):110.

Neuman B. (1980). The Betty Neuman health-care systems model: a total person approach to patient problems. In *Conceptual Models for Nursing Practice*, 2nd edn (Riehl J.P., Roy C., eds.) pp. 119–134. New York: Appleton-Century-Crofts.

Nursing Development Conference Group (NDCG) (1973). *Concept Formalisation in Nursing*, 2nd edn. Boston: Little, Brown.

Nuttall P. (1975). The need. In *New Horizons in Clinical Nursing* pp. 3–4. London: Royal College of Nursing.

Orem D. (1980). *Nursing: Concepts of Practice*. New York: McGraw Hill.

Ottoway R.M. (1976). A change of strategy to implement new norms, new style and new environment in the work organisation. *Personnel Review;* **5**(1):13.

Pembrey S. (1980). *The Ward Sister — Key to Nursing*. London: Royal College of Nursing.

Peplau H.E. (1969). Professional closeness. *Nursing Forum*; **8**:4.

Phaneuf M. (1976). *The Nursing Audit*. New York: Appleton-Century-Crofts.

Poirer B. (1975). Loeb Center — what nursing can and should be. *The American Nurse;* **7**(1):5.

Powers M.J. (1976). The unification model in nursing. *Nursing Outlook;* **24**:8.

Report of the Committee on Nursing (Briggs Committee; 1972). *Great Britain, Parliament*. London: HMSO.

Riehl J.P. (1980). The Riehl interaction model. In *Conceptual Models for Nursing Practice* (Riehl J.P., Roy C., eds.) pp. 350–356. New York: Appleton-Century-Crofts.

Riehl J.P., Roy C. (1980). *Conceptual Models for Nursing Practice*. New York: Appleton-Century-Crofts.

Rines A., Montag M. (1976). *Nursing Concepts and Nursing Care*. New York: Wiley.

Rogers M.E. (1980). Nursing: a science of unitary man. In *Conceptual Models for Nursing Practice* (Riehl J.P., Roy C., eds.) pp. 329–338. New York: Appleton-Century-Crofts.

Roper N. (1976). *Clinical Experience in Nurse Education*. Edinburgh: Churchill Livingstone.

Roper N. (1979). Nursing based on a model of living. In *Readings in Nursing* (Colledge M.M., Jones D., eds.) pp. 81–91. Edinburgh: Churchill Livingstone.

Roper N., Logan W.W., Tierney A.J. (1980). *The Elements of Nursing*. Edinburgh: Churchill Livingstone.

Roy C. (1980). The Roy adaptation model. In *Conceptual Models for Nursing Practice* (Riehl J.P., Roy C., eds.) pp. 179–188. New York: Appleton-Century-Crofts.

Royal College of Nursing (1971). *Evidence to the Committee on Nursing*. London: Royal College of Nursing.

Royal College of Nursing (1975). *New Horizons in Clinical Nursing*. London: Royal College of Nursing.

Royal College of Nursing (1979). *Discussion Paper of the Working Party of a Clinical Career Structure for Nurses*. London: Royal College of Nursing.

Royal College of Nursing (1981). *Towards Standards*. London: Royal College of Nursing.

Royal Commission on the National Health Service. Report (1979). London: HMSO.

Salmon Committee (1966). *Great Britain, Ministry of Health*. Report of the Committee on the Senior Nursing Staff Structure. London: HMSO.

Schaffrath W.B. (1978). Commission leads way to joint practice for nurses and physicians. *Hospitals;* **52**(14):78.

Schmadl J.C. (1979). Quality assurance: examination of the concept. *Nursing Outlook;* **27**:7.

Schweer J.E. (1972). *Creative Teaching in Clinical Nursing*. St Louis, Miss: C.V. Mosby.

Sheahan D. (1972). The game of the name— nurse professional and nurse technician. *Nursing Outlook;* **20**:440.

Silver M.A. (1980). *The Nurse Consultant Clinician: an Advanced Clinical Role in Paediatric Nursing*. Unpublished MSc Thesis. Manchester: Department of Nursing: University of Manchester.

Sjoberg K. (1968). *Patient Classification Study*. Saskatoon: University of Saskatchewan.

Sjoberg K., Bicknell P. (1969). *A Pilot Study to Implement and Evaluate the Unit Assignment System*. Saskatoon: University of Saskatchewan.

Sjoberg K., Heieren, E.L. and Jackson, M.R. (1971). Unit assignment: a patient centered system. *Nursing Clinics of North America;* **6**:2.

Stein L. (1978). The doctor–nurse game. In *Readings in the Sociology of Nursing* (Dingwall R., McIntosh J., eds.) pp. 107–117. Edinburgh: Churchill Livingstone.

Stockwell P. (1972). *The Unpopular Patient*. London: Royal College of Nursing.

Szasz T.S. (1972). *The Myth of Mental Illness*. St Albans: Paladin.

Theis C., Harrington H. (1968). Three factors that affect practice—communications, assignments, attitudes. *American Journal of Nursing;* **68**(8):1478.

Tiffany C.H. (1977). *Nursing Organisational Structure and the Real Goals of Hospitals.* Unpublished PhD Thesis. Indiana University.

Tobin H.M., Wise P.S.Y., Hull P.K. (1974). *The Process of Staff Development.* St Louis, Miss: C.V. Mosby.

Travelbee J. (1971). *Interpersonal Aspects of Nursing.* Philadelphia: F.A. Davis.

Treece E.W., Treece J.W. (1977). *Elements of Research in Nursing.* St Louis, Miss: C.V. Mosby.

Tyler L. (1965). *The Psychology of Human Differences.* New York: Appleton-Century-Crofts.

Van Dersal W. (1974). *The Successful Supervisor in Government and Business.* London: Harper & Row.

Wandelt M., Ager J. (1974). *Quality Patient Care Scale.* New York: Appleton-Century-Crofts.

Weber M. (1947). *The Theory of Social and Economic Organisation.* New York: Appleton-Century-Crofts.

Wiedenbach E. (1964). *Clinical Nursing.* New York: Springer.

Wilson J. (1972). *Philosophy and Educational Research.* Windsor: National Foundation for Educational Research in England and Wales.

Wolford H.G. (1964). Complemental nursing care. *Nursing Forum;* **3**:8.

Wright L. (1974). *Bowel Function in Hospital Patients.* London: Royal College of Nursing.

Yura H., Walsh M.B. (1973). *The Nursing Process.* New York: Appleton-Century-Crofts.

Zimmer M.J. (1980). A nursing service administration perspective. *Nursing Research;* **29**:2.

Zola I.R. (1975). Medicine as an institution of social control. In *A Sociology of Medical Practice* (Cox C., Mead A., eds.) pp. 170–185. London: Collier Macmillan.

Zornow R.A. (1977). A curriculum model for the expanded role. *Nursing Outlook;* **25**(1):43.

Index

108

JOCELY   ies
of 1990 a   has
co-edited   he
Best Stage   us,
Inc., 1991)   es:
A Sourcebo

LIBREX —

GREGORY MOSHER is the Director of the Lincoln Center Theater
in New York City.

i

Other Books for Actors from Smith and Kraus

The Best Men's Stage Monologues of 1990
    edited by Jocelyn Beard

The Best Women's Stage Monologues of 1990
    edited by Jocelyn Beard

Street Talk: Character Monologues for Actors
    by Glenn Alterman

Great Scenes for Young Actors from the Stage
    Craig Slaight and Jack Sharrar, editors

The Best Stage Scenes for Men from the 1980's
    edited by Jocelyn A. Beard and Kristin Graham

The Best Stage Scenes for Women from the 1980's
    edited by Jocelyn A. Beard and Kristin Graham

One Hundred Women's Stage Monologues from the 1980's
    edited by Jocelyn A. Beard

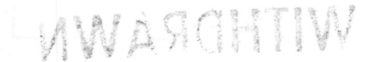

ONE HUNDRED
MEN'S STAGE
MONOLOGUES
FROM THE 1980'S

Edited by
Jocelyn A. Beard

SK
A Smith and Kraus Book

A Smith and Kraus Book
Published by Smith and Kraus, Inc.

Cover design by David Wise
Text design by Jeannette Champagne

First Edition: July 1991
10 9 8 7 6 5 4

Publisher's Cataloging in Publication
(Prepared by Quality Books Inc.)

One hundred men's stage monologues from the 1980's / edited by Jocelyn
A. Beard. --
  p. cm.
  Includes bibliographical references.
  ISBN 0-9622722-4-8
  1. Monologues. 2. Acting--Auditions. I. Beard, Jocelyn A.,
1955-

PN2080   808.8245
                                    91-61810
                                    MARC

Smith and Kraus, Inc.
177 Lyme Road, Hanover, NH 03755
www.smithkraus.com

ACKNOWLEDGMENTS

Grateful thanks to the playwrights.

CONTENTS

CONTENTS

CONTENTS

CONTENTS

x

CONTENTS

CONTENTS

FOREWORD

The 80's was a decade of great social and political transition. As society finally managed to set aside the issues of the 60's and 70's, it found itself straddling the vast technological, social and political gaps that would eventually lead us into the 1990's.

Playwrights were especially challenged during this time, and the mens' characters they created are rich and varied. Included in this collection are men like Peter, who teaches us about the tragedy of AIDS and its influence on mens' relationships in Richard Greenberg's *Eastern Standard*; a sad tale of lovers meeting too late in life. The legacy of southern racism helped Jane Martin to create the scary monster, Ryman in *Coups/Clucks*.

As you can see, theater from the 80's provides men with fantastic challenges and opportunities. Mens' roles became increasingly complex during this time of New Age vs. Old Age. Gone, for example, is the simplistic family man of the 70's, as can be seen in Donald Margulies' devastating treatise on the disintegration of the family: *The Loman Family Picnic*. On the other hand, men have newly-gained insight into women during this time as the intrepid Johnny pursues wounded Frankie in Terrence McNally's *Frankie and Johnny in the Clair de Lune*.

The drama of international events helped to provide men with daring new roles as we can see in such works as Athol Fugard's cry against apartheid, *My Children! My Africa!*. *Kissing the Pope*, Nick Darke's tale of young Contras in Nicaragua provide the actor with an opportunity to explore the psyche of young men motivated by fear, ignorance and a lust for violence. Back on the home front, the murders of Harvey Milk and George Moscone in San Francisco brought the ugly specter of homophobia to national attention and gave playwright Emily Mann the inspiration to write *Execution of Justice*.

The 80's had a lighter side, thank goodness, and those of you searching for comic material will be delighted by the wonderfully absurd characters created by Christopher Durang in *Laughing Wild*.

If anything, the 80's were complete. From romance (*Archangels*

FOREWORD

Don't Play Pinball) to historical fantasy (*After Aida*) virtually every genre of theater was explored and is subsequently contained herein. Roles for Hispanics, Asian Americans, and African Americans are included, and it is this editor's hope that these selections will continue to increase and improve as time goes on.

Reading through theater from the 80's was sometimes exhausting and painful but immensely satisfying in the end. This was surely a time of artistic watershed that has provided men with classic roles which I urge you to exploit as best you can. Take a deep breath, and keep reading!

—Jocelyn A. Beard
Patterson, NY
May, 1991

INTRODUCTION

One fine day when I was a young director I bumped into a wise and famous and successful friend in the same occupation. We hadn't seen each other for a while and I suggested coffee. He said that he was off to audition two actors and could see me in three hours for lunch. Didn't three hours seem a little <u>excessive</u>, I wondered? "Look," said the wise and successful and famous director, "I'm about to spend 18 months with these people. A morning isn't very much time." My wise <u>etcetera</u> friend, his show, and the two actors won every award but the Heisman Trophy that year, and this brief episode made a lasting impression.

Elia Kazan wrote that he didn't like auditions very much, and that he could learn more about someone by taking a walk together in the park. I figure that he's not alone in disliking and distrusting auditions. And most of you reading this book are probably a ways off from having the kind of audition or meeting that rates more than a quick impression. But even two minute pieces can lead, eventually, to work. They are how most of us got started, and they are here to stay.

At some point, you'll audition by reading from the play. After that, if you are lucky, your work will be known well enough that you'll just be invited to join the company. (Become a movie star and you can audition the director.) In each case, the idea is the same. Someone—a director, or coach, or teacher, or producer, or agent—is considering making a substantial commitment to you. These people have two questions: 1. Can you serve the goal of the production? 2. Will the process be stimulating for both parties? And, believe it or not, people who audition have usually learned how to discover a lot in five minutes.

So how do you choose an audition piece? Two simple rules, I think. Pick something you love, because you are going to live with it even in your dreams. And choose something that is appropriate to your general age and disposition. Each of us has a Stanley Kowalski and a Blanche DuBois inside us. That is what makes them classic characters. But very few of us are seen to our best advantage auditioning in those roles.

Now that you've chosen, how to you prepare? Obviously this question can't be answered in a whole book, much less an introduction to one, but the thing to remember is that the rules of auditioning are the same as the rules of acting. It is your job, in Stanislavski's phrase, "to live truthfully under imaginary circumstances." If you like showy, artificial acting, then by all means emulate it. But if telling the truth in a simple way is your idea of a good work (as it is mine), that's what you must do at your audition.

As we know, the best way to do that is to choose a verb for your speech. Use the playwright's words to <u>do</u> something: to "ridicule", to "implore", to "seduce", to "defend my position". This verb comes from the intention of the scene, of course, not from the text, which merely provides the clues. "What's your sign?" is not generally considered to be a scientific inquiry.

The other issue is to whom the monologue or speech is addressed. "Persuading" your mother to borrow the car for the weekend is different than "persuading" a cop not to give you a ticket. The question of the addressee is the tricky thing, because good acting requires that you put your attention on the other actor, and what you don't have with a prepared monologue is another actor. In most of the speeches in this book you are sharing the stage with someone who happens not to be speaking at the moment. It's a scene, even if you have all the lines. This isn't the same as Hamlet having a nice chat with himself, but it is what happens every day. So preparing with someone is an excellent idea.

A question everyone seems to have is: Should I look at the person auditioning? The answer is: I don't know. Some people like it. Some hate it. Some like being asked. Some don't. I don't mind being asked, and my answer is "no." I have enough to do watching you without having to silently improvise with you. So my suggestion is go with what seems comfortable for the speech and be ready to switch.

INTRODUCTION

You aren't in control of most of what happens in the audition, from the quality of the coffee they're drinking to how late they're running. But they do want you to be good. They're auditioning you because they are looking for someone wonderful and in your five minutes, hundreds of hours of work are about to be revealed. As Hamlet says, "The readiness is all". So be ready.

As a young actor, what you have is a lot of time. So use it. Practice singing. Learn to dance. Memorize ten lines of Shakespeare a day. Lose the eight pounds you've been meaning to lose. Have six monologues ready. And understand that there is all the difference in the world between the actor who can do a passable dance combination and the one who says he "moves well." And that the person who has a good voice and a bouquet of dialects will always beat out the person who claims to have "a good ear."

A few final thoughts. It never hurts to know who's in the room before you go in. It's okay to be personal, since no director ever minded hearing that someone saw, let alone liked, a show. But don't expect, or initiate, a discussion. If you are auditioning for a new play, an expression of enthusiasm for the work is appreciated and appropriate. New plays are hard, and directors are looking for allies as well as colleagues.

So here you are, on the verge of creating something unique in the theater, simply by being you. Remember that there is no other person like you. Work on your craft so that that person can be revealed. Serve the playwright's intentions. Be true to your principles and your pals. And have a wonderful life in the theater.

—Gregory Mosher
Director
Lincoln Center Theater
New York, New York

ONE HUNDRED
MEN'S STAGE
MONOLOGUES
FROM THE 1980'S

MOUNTAIN
by Douglas Scott
The mind of a dying man - January 19, 1980 - William (30-40)

Supreme Court Justice William O. Douglas authored the decision
that assures a Constitutional right to privacy among many others.
The great man is dying and is here transformed in his mind into
his younger self.

DOUGLAS: Yes! I'm dying! *(A pause. With each beat, Douglas
gradually more vigorous, in charge.)* But that's not the *last* thing
I'm gonna do. I've planned my own *funeral.* And it's going to
shake up that damn Establishment. They're going to bury me at
Arlington—got the spot all picked: not far from Jack Kennedy—and
only twenty feet from Oliver Wendell Holmes. And there I'll be—
among all those Generals and Secretaries of Defense. And you
know what my tombstone is going to say? "William O. Douglas:
Private, United States Army." *(Cackles.)* And for the funeral, I'll
have the U.S. Army Chorus sing, "Shall We Gather At The River."
Right? And just when they're thinking that at the end, Bill Douglas
got all soft, I'm gonna have that Army Chorus hit 'em with a song
by Woody Guthrie: "This Land is Your Land"! By God, I just wish
John Foster Dulles could be there. The blood would drain right out
of that Episcopalian face. *(Laughs. Surprised at himself, calling
offstage.)* Tell those doctors I've decided not to die! *(To audience.)*
They're probably all Republicans! Oh, I gotta admit it: not *every*
Republican is like John Foster Dulles. Some of the bastards actually
have a sense of humor. Did'ja hear what Bob Dole called our last
three Presidents—Carter, Ford, and Nixon? Called 'em "See No
Evil." "Hear No Evil." And... "Evil"! Well, and a lot of these
Democrats today. They're no bargain either. Bunch of
weathervanes. Pisses me off. Some of those fellows think they're
gonna be more conservative than a Republican. Can't be done.
Like trying to be more ugly than a spider. You got to face the fact:
Republicans and spiders have conservative and ugly *all locked up!*
(He laughs happily.) I'm feeling better! These goddam doctors

1

won't let me do *any*thing. Everything's "dangerous." Well shit, of *course* it is. *Life* is dangerous. If you *live* it! *(Calls offstage.)* And I've decided to *live*! Right up to the Bicentennials! The *real* ones. Not that thing that Gerald Ford had in Seventy-Six—for the Revolution. Any fool country can have a revolution. But what *this* nation obtained was our Constitution and our Bill of Rights! They give life and protection to the minorities. And by that, I mean *all* of us. Every man and woman is a minority of one. And he and she, if it comes to that, must have the right to stand up to the full and awesome majesty of this Government, and say—*unafraid*: "Here is this small, humble area that is my life. And it *is mine*. So you, United States of America, get off my back!"

THE PINK STUDIO
by Jane Anderson
France - Early 20th century - Henri (40-50)

This play is a series of vignettes from the life of artist Henri Matisse. Each scene uses as its background, a particular painting of Matisse. Here, Henri describes painting a prostitute.

(Henri is standing in front of his painting, NUDE WITH TAMBOURINE.)

HENRI: I had to pay Nicole the fee for "three screws", as she put it, in order to get her to pose for me. She made me close the shutters halfway so it wasn't too bright. She pulled off her robe. There were purple bruises all up and down her arms and legs. "One of my clients is in love with me," she said, "and since he can't have me, he beats me." I was appalled. "This has to stop," I said. "No one can make it stop," she said, "because I'm in love with him too." She showed me a tambourine that he had given her. The skin of the drum looked as bruised as Nicole. "Gerard is with a Spanish band," she said. "He beats the tambourine while he sings about me. That is how he expresses himself. That is his art." This made me furious. "He's a monster," I said, "Beating a woman has nothing to do with art!" I was determined to show her how gently and respectfully a true artist works. I posed her in the shape of a question mark, a beautiful, classic pose. I painted out her bruises and emphasized the pattern in an oriental rug that was on the floor. I finished the painting in about an hour and a half and I was very pleased with the result. I showed it to Nicole. "Nicole," I said, "do you see what an artist can do when he uses his eyes instead of his fists?" "Yes," she said, "you make something pretty without any balls." "What do you mean, it has no balls?" I said. "Passion," she said. "Gerard has passion." Then she told me to leave so she could take a nap. I packed up my paints and left, feeling like a perfect ass. When I got back to the hotel, Claudine wasn't there. There was only a message at the desk: "I have gone out. Don't wait up for me. As always, Claudine." I thought, well fine, she's

3

getting back at me for being late. I deserve it. When it got to be past midnight, I rang the police. When I showed them the note they laughed and said if they saw her, they'd send her home early. I tried to go to bed but of course I couldn't sleep. Around about dawn, I took out the painting of Nicole. The more I looked at it, the more I wanted to kick it in. Instead, I loaded up my palette and added what I knew had to be there—the wretched tambourine. It had a red stripe around the rim and I thought, "what the hell," and let the color bleed onto the floor. I made it red, everything red. I was all set to take it back and show it to the whore: "Is this passionate enough for you?! LOOK AT THIS! IS THIS PASSIONATE ENOUGH FOR YOU?!

(A bell rings.)

And then the bell rang. It was the concierge. Claudine was in the lobby.

RACING DEMON
by David Hare
London - Present - Streaky (40-50)

The Rev. Donald "Streaky" Bacon has watched while his church
is divided into two camps by the older vicar and an idealistic
young priest. After several cocktails, Streaky shares some of his
thoughts with God.

STREAKY: Drunk, Lord, drunk.

And blissfully happy. Can't help it. Love this job. Love my
work. Look at other people in total bewilderment. I got to drink at
the Savoy. It was wonderful. It's all wonderful. Why can't people
enjoy what they have?

Is it just a matter of temperament? I mean, I'm a happy
priest. Always have been. Ever since I got my first job as curate
as St Anselm's, Cheam, because they needed a light tenor for the
parochial Gilbert and Sullivan society. Matins, a sung Eucharist,
two Evensongs and *Iolanthe* five nights a week.

It was bliss. I loved it. I tried to start it here. But there's
something deep in the Jamaican character that can't find its
way through *The Pirates of Penzance*. It's still bliss, though. They
are blissful people. Once a year we take the coach to the sea. On
the way down we have the rum and the curried goat. Lord, there is
no end to your goodness. Then we have rum and curried goat on
the way back.

Lord, I have no theology. Can't do it. By my bed, there's a
pile of paperbacks called *The Meaning of Meaning*, and *How to Ask
Why*. They've been there for years. The whole thing's so clear.
He's there. In people's happiness. Tonight, in the taste of that
drink. Or the love of my friends. The whole thing's so simple.
Infinitely loving.

Why do people find it so hard?

BACK STREET MAMMY
by Trish Cooke
London - Present - Skolar (40-50)

Skolar is the domineering and abusive patriarch of a West Indian
family that has moved to England in search of a better life.
When Skolar encounters Jacko, an old friend, he reveals his
over-protective feelings for his youngest daughter.

SKOLAR: [You raise up me hat you don't see how me head white
already. *(Stuups.)* Jacko man...life eh.

I see... *(Pause.)*] I see me las' chil' turn woman on me. Think
she can treat my house how she want. Bring man at all hours. All
night I hear dem humph humph on me hire purchase sofa...makin'
noise in me head all night. And is me las' girl Jacko. She have
brains dat one. She me las' girl, me las' hope to make me know I
didn't come to dis damn place for nothing... All night Jacko I
hearing de spring in me sofa and me baby going away from me man.
And it was de firs' time, de firs' time in the line of girl chil' I have
there, the firs' time I stay in me bed, hol' onto de sheet and try and
block out de noise. De firs' time I never hol' a knife to his throat
and run de likkle skunt outta me house, outta me daughter...de firs'
time Jacko... And you know why man...you know why? Cos I was
scared. I was scared, and wouldn't I be a sick man if it *was* true
what Maria say mm? Dat I was jealous of de man lying on me sofa
wid me daughter. Jealous of de man who taste firs'.

(He looks at JACKO hard.)

Now wouldn't I be a sick man?

[JACKO *(trying to avoid the conclusion of the conversation)*: Man
is long time since I see you daughter; she real pretty. You should
be proud...]

SKOLAR: Yes...I would be a sick man. You know what I saying
enn it Jacko. It like a burning right in you stomach, right in de pit
of you stomach... Like when you have a cake dat don't cut yet and
somebody come in de night and take piece...when somebody cut de
cake before your birthday den de birthday spoil ne true. Well is that
what I talking.

6

THE END OF I
from Sex and Death
by Diana Amsterdam
Brooklyn - Present - Jerome (30's)

Jerome is facing a mid-life crisis along with a touch of death anxiety brought on by the premature death of his friend in a motorcycle accident. Tortured by his fear of nothingness, Jerome is unable to sleep. He wakes his wife and confides his fears.

JEROME: What is death?

[ALICE: We'll figure it out in the morning.]

JEROME: You always say that. You always say we'll figure it out in the morning, but how will we figure it out? Do you know how to figure it out? I've been trying for three weeks to figure it out, and I can't figure anything out. I can't figure a damn thing out. Did it ever occur to you that death could be nothing? Nothing, Alice. Nothing. Nothing. Nothing. Death could be nothing. Nothing, Alice. Death could be absolutely nothing. Can you figure out nothing? Can you? Can you figure out nothing? Can you find nothing? Can you experience nothing? Can you *be* nothing? Try to *be* nothing. Go ahead, Alice. I dare you. Try it. *(ALICE is asleep.)* Try it. Try to be nothing. Try it. Just try it, Alice. Just try it. Just try it for one minute. For one second. Try it. Just try to *be* nothing. Not just nothing, nothingness. Try to be nothingness for one minute. For one second. Absolutely nothing. I don't mean something. I don't mean wake-up-in-a-few-hours. I mean nothing. Nothing. No thing, nothing. No feel. No smell. No taste. No see. No nothing. No nothing. No me. No I. No I. *(HE bolts upright, extremely agitated.)* Alice. Alice. *(HE shakes HER awake.)*

[ALICE: Come here, darling.]

JEROME: No! Don't tempt me! You fall into a woman's arms you can't even begin to understand nothing, nothing just disappears, nothing just evaporates, all around you there's something,

THE END OF I

something, something. Women are very dangerous, Alice. *(ALICE is asleep.)* Women make you believe that you're going to live forever. And you're not going to live forever. You're going to die! Die! Die! Die! Die! Stay away from me, Alice! Alice. Alice! Oh God, I love you, I love you Alice, I love you. I love you. I love you. I love you. I love you and I love our daughters. I love their eyes, I love their hair, I love their little fingernails. I love their tiny shoes. I love those little sheets you bought them, the ones with the butterflies. *(Notices the sheet under him.)* I love this sheet. I love this sheet! *(Rubs the sheet.)* I don't want to leave this sheet! I don't want to! I love it! I love this sheet! I don't want to! Would it go on without me? Could it go on without me? Could it? Would it? Where would I be? Where's Marty, Alice? What happened to Marty? Where did he go? One minute he was riding his motorcycle, zooming with the wind on his face more alive that at any other time except inside a woman and the next minute, blotto! Gone! Zap! Disappeared! *People disappear off this planet, Alice. All the time.* Can't you save me? Can't your love save me? Save me, Alice, save me!

A FEW GOOD MEN
by Aaron Sorkin
Washington, DC - Summer, 1986 - Jessep (40-50)

This Marine Lt. Colonel is loyal to the Corps above all other
things. When one of his men dies as a result of a "Code Red"—
an unofficial act of internal discipline—Jessep finds himself
giving testimony at the courtmarshall of the two men charged
with the crime. When he is asked to tell the truth about "Code
Red", he explodes with anger, revealing his fanatical devotion
to the Corps.

JESSEP: Captain, for the past month, this man has attempted to put
the Marine Corps on trial. I think somebody sure as hell better
address this question or people are liable to start listening to him.
[KAFFEE: Why is it impossible—?]
[JESSEP: Because you can't handle it, son. You can't handle the
truth. You can't handle the sad but historic reality.]
[KAFFEE: What reality are you referring to, Colonel?]
JESSEP: We live in a world that has walls. And those walls have
to be guarded by men with guns. Who's gonna do it? You? *(To
Sam.)* You, Lt. Weinberg? I have a greater responsibility than you
can possibly fathom. You weep for Santiago, and you curse the
Marines. You have that luxury. The luxury of the blind. The
luxury of not knowing what I know: That Santiago's death, while
tragic, probably saved lives. And my existence, while grotesque and
incomprehensible to you...saves lives. You can't handle it. Because
deep down, in places you don't talk about, you *want* me on that
wall. You need me there. We use words like honor, code, loyalty.
We use these words as a backbone to a life spent defending
something. You use them as a punchline. I have neither the time
nor the inclination to explain myself to a man who rises and sleeps
under the blanket of the very freedom I provide, then questions the
manner in which I provide it. I'd prefer you just said thank you and
went on your way. Otherwise, I'd suggest you pick up a weapon
and stand a post. Either way. I don't give a damn what you think
you're entitled to.

9

FIGHTING LIGHT
by Greg Zittel
Verona, New Jersey - 1930's - Al Hoffman (20's)

Al Hoffman has been set up on a blind date with Molly Farrell, a firey young woman with a mind of her own. When their initial encounter goes poorly, an angered and bemused Al rails against women to his friend, Marty.

AL: Well you saw her. There. Look. See? Ain't they beautiful? Ain't it all terrific? They get all dolled up like for you and me. You dunce, this was your idea, you got me up here. I don't need to be running around up here where they dodge the chickens to have a good time. This monkey business ain't for me. You give in now, you're trapped. *(Sits in wicker chair.)* They trap you. They get their paws wrapped around your neck and they squeeze the life right out of you. They make it like there's bars around you. They slam the gate shut and you do time. You don't live no more. You do time. They choke the air right out of you. Squeezing just like they're doing now dammit and the only way to fight it is to stand against it. Don't let it get you. Marty, come with me and let's make it out of here while we still got our respect. Come on, goddammit, are you with me?

GHETTO
by Joshua Sobol
in a version by David Lan
Vilna, Lithuania - 1939-1943 - Weiskopf (40-50)

A Jew interred in the ghettos at Vilna, Weiskopf constantly
strives to make the best of things. Here, the entrepeneaurial
Weiskopf admonsishes the director of the ghetto's theater group
for using the stage to complain about their situation.

WEISKOPF: Times are hard? So times are hard. When did Jews
have it easy? You tell me. Suffering makes us strong, gives us
power. Look at me. I could stand and cry. I've got good reason.
Before the war I had a drapery. The war came. So they pushed me
in here. My shop? *Kaput!* Could I cry? And how! But did I?

I said to myself: why do they call you Weiskopf? Wise Kopf.
So I took my wise Jewish kopf and I said: the shop you lost. Will
crying bring it back? My arse. If you lose your head as well,
you're done for. Nothing else can save you. And that they can't
take, not as long as you're alive.

Next I looked around. Walls. A ghetto. I'm closed in. Can I
find an opening? Where? I found it! Before the war I was what?
A miserable textile worker. Now? I'm managing a tailor's
workshop. In the whole region it's number one. Two months and
this head's taken me so far! I've got a hundred and fifty Jews
working under me. One hundred and fifty! The Germans place
their orders, buy my clothes. It's a gigantic operation!

Each day it's getting bigger. The sun rises, my income rises
too. And I don't sit on it. My hands are open! If I make a
donation to a cause, I give at least five thousand. I'm generous.
And I don't hide it. Why should I? Let everyone see and hear. I
want the world to know. I'm not ashamed! I make a living and I
let others live. Hundreds of others!

Take my example, boys and girls. I'm nothing special. We
Jews have talent, more than any other people. If more of us did
what I do and stop that whining and complaining, this ghetto would
be productive. The Germans would need us! We'd be an asset.
Could they get by without us? No! That way we'd survive!

11

INCOMMUNICADO
by Tom Dulack
Pisa, Italy - 1945 - Ezra Pound (50's)

The US Army has detained expatriate poet, Ezra Pound, in Italy at the close of the second World War. Pound stands charged with treason and here reveals his sardonic nature as he taunts the MP assigned to guard him.

POUND: I think there must be some mistake. I don't belong here. The name is Pound. P.O.U.N.D. As in Of Flesh. Poet. A.K.A., also know as, The Great Bass. *Il Miglior Fabbro*, Gospel according to Eliot. I'm sure it's a procedural matter, a legal technicality, clear it up in no time. If I could just see a lawyer, clear it up in no time, count on it, bet on it. *(Calling.)* Hey, you! Hey, Buck! Hey, Kingfish! Hey, Rochester! I've got my rights, you hear me, boy? You can't execute a man without a trial and unless things changed since I been out of the country, you can't have a trial without letting me consult with an advocate. Even the United States Army can't execute an American citizen without providing him with legal counsel. *(The MP returns, silent, big, all menace and institutional brutality. He takes up a position to one side of the cage and does not look at Pound. In a shift, fearing another water assault.)* Anyway, at least a pencil and a scrap of paper. You see, I don't have any writing implements. None of the tools of my trade. What do you say, Sergeant? Think you could work on some paper and a couple pencil stubs for Ole Ez? Problem is, I've got no time, Sergeant. And there's so much to do. Maybe you can't appreciate that a man on death row can have a need to do things. But there's all the more reason, being on death row. I have so much still to say, so much imagining to do. See? That's my job. Imagining. It's what I do... *(A siren erupts. The MP gives a start, tenses but doesn't move. There are shouts in the distance, whistles. A searchlight explodes across the yard sweeping back and forth. There is the sound of large dogs barking. Then short bursts of machine gun fire. After which, silence.)* Anybody ever make it over the

INCOMMUNICADO

wall, Jim? Anybody ever make it out of here in one piece? To the best of your—using a term loosely—knowledge? *(The MP doesn't answer. He moves around the cage, takes up a position on the other side. He conveys the impression that he is somehow tentative, curious even, though very hostile.)* Sneaking admiration, though, admit it. For the gallantry. The sheer desperate gallantry of the attempt. Desperate men. You ever think of it that way, Jim? You're in a fair way to become an authority on the inner workings of the souls of desperate men. Could write a book some day, if you could write, hey, Jim? Ever get that shameful itch in your loins? Ever wonder what it's *like*, Jim? Ever lie there at night dreaming about plunging your bad old utensil into that forbidden honeypot? Your prehensile utensil? Hey, Jim? You be careful. Keep your pants buttoned up, Jim. Look where writing got *me*. It's where it gets all of us. Five minutes of pleasure and then a lifetime of clap, take my word. My Word! My words. What do you say, Jim? You can't shoot a man without first he writes a last will and testament.

[MP: You ain't supposed to talk! You got no privileges. You're bein' held incommunicado and that means you ain't supposed to talk. It's against the rules for you to talk!]

POUND: It's a question of velocity. I've lived my life at a tremendous velocity, a tremendous intellectual velocity. My brain *spins*, Jim, it whirls, it careens. The inside of my skull is a regular velodrome. There's a lot of centrifugal pressure that needs to be relieved. I gotta formulate me some words, friend, I gotta write, you gotta let me write, else I'm going to die.

13

INÉS DE CASTRO
by John Clifford
Portugal - 14th Century - King (50's)

During a war with Spain, the King of Portugal orders the execution of his son's Spanish consort and her children. The old man knows that he has commited a great sin and despairs, for his own death is near.

KING: I keep having dreams. People keep knocking on the door. And I have to open it. I say, it isn't right, I'm the king. I shouldn't have to do this. I'm the king! But they take no notice. They just keep filing in. Hundreds of them. Hundreds. People with their wounds. All festering. Horrible. Horrible. It was a fair fight, I tell them. Entirely fair. Nothing personal. Just go away. Go away! But there's more of them. More. And more. And more.

She never comes. Not Inés. Never. She knows better. It had to happen. I've no regrets. None. None at all.

I'm walking down a passage. It's very long. There are so many doors. I'm trying to open them but I've thrown away the keys. I'm naked and afraid. There's a man further up coming after me. I'm looking for some armour. I try all the doors. But I can't get in. I can't get in. I'm naked. Then I look down. My armour has become my skin.

I'm in a dried-up river bed. My feet raise clouds of dust. A voice says 'Cross' and I start to try. But I don't know the way. I don't know which is forward, which is back. I try to move but my legs don't work. I try to move but I'm getting buried. I'm getting buried in the sand...

And then I'm by a canyon, standing by this great enormous hole. It's very deep, and black. Quite black. I know it has no end. And all the river's pouring into it. And I think 'So that's where all the water goes.' And the voice says 'Now walk. Go across.' And then my feet start moving. And then I know. Then I know I've died.

KISSING THE POPE
by Nick Darke
Honduras - Present - Sanchez (17)

This young Nicaraguan has been made into a brutal killer by his training at the Contra base in Honduras. After a devastating run-in with the Sandanistas, Sanchez flees over the mountains to Hounduras, taking Emilio—a young boy whose father he has viciously tortured and murdered—with him. As they huddle next to a portable cooking-stove, Sanchez boasts to Emilio of his ability to kill and lectures on the state of the world, as he understands it.

SANCHEZ: Always bivouac on top of a mountain. You're above the enemy and you gotta downhill start in the morning. *(Taps his forehead.)* Psychological see?
(Exit SANCHEZ.)
(EMILIO is on his back with his haversack beneath him. He is too tired to get up. He jerks himself over onto his side.)
(Enter SANCHEZ with two yucca roots.)
Eat yucca?
(SANCHEZ unhooks his water canteen from his belt and washes the yucca. He slings a yucca to EMILIO and starts chewing his. He looks around him, reconnoitring.)
Old cattle trail this. Can't light a fire yet. You think you're safe and they grow up out the ground in front of you, Sandinistas, like ghosts.
(He manhandles EMILIO onto his front and unstraps his rolled up groundsheet and poncho-liner.)
Leave mosta this behind tomorrer. Travel light the last day.
(He hikes EMILIO up onto his knees.)
(EMILIO unbuckles his harness, lets slip the haversack and collapses to the ground.)
(SANCHEZ unpacks his haversack. He unclips a torch from his uniform breast and places it close by. He takes an optimus stove from his haversack. Then he takes a tin of baked beans, two

15

aluminium hash-cans, tin-opener, spoons and lighter. He opens the beans and starts cooking.)

(He is speaking whilst unpacking.)

SANCHEZ: We're moving into big-unit warfare now we've got the numbers. Upper echelon's planning an offensive on Ocotal in the very near future. We're putting three thousand men into Ocotal. Clear a landing strip and declare the town a liberated area. So the non-aligned countries like NATO can send us aid direct to Ocotal. From there we free the north-eastern sector, march south, and liberate Managua. After that we take a shower. Hah! *(He laughs.)*

(Howler monkeys shriek.)

Fulla Russians, Managua. Fulla Cubans. Know what they do? They piss in hypodermics and inject the babies with it. Then they bite the babies heads off as they're dying. They cut off men's balls and fry 'em. Cubans go to war over a man's balls to eat. Castro eats 'em by the cart-load. Since he quit cigars Cuba's fulla eunuchs. The Sandinistas force their women to eat their own afterbirth to make 'em fecund. Disgusts me. The priests are forced to eat their own shit and all the churches used as brothels.

(The beans are cooking. SANCHEZ eats his yucca. EMILIO is too tired to eat.)

SANCHEZ: Come on. Eat your yucca.

(EMILIO takes a bite.)

SANCHEZ: Fuck knows what we're gonna find when we take Managua. The misery.

(The beans are nearly ready. SANCHEZ stirs them.)

They'll be mobilising when we get back, for Ocotal. But you and me won't be going. I'll make sure a that. 'Cos Ocotal's gonna be a bloodbath whoever wins. Thass why we gotta make fuckin' sure I get two stripes, a citation and my picture in the *Miami Herald*. So we get a special op' a long way from Ocotal. With me?

(SANCHEZ takes the pan off the stove and hands it to EMILIO. EMILIO takes the beans.)

Hot enough for ya?

KISSING THE POPE

(EMILIO nods and starts to eat slowly. SANCHEZ starts to cook his beans.)

SANCHEZ: I'll have to dream up a nom de guerre for the *Miami Herald*.

(He stirs his beans.)

I take the Pope with me wherever I go 'cos I'm killin' for the Pope. Thass the first thing they tell you at Camp. You gotta have a reason and you gotta know why. Then they show you how. First thing you do is close-quarter combat with an Irish chap called El Chino. 'Cos to kill with one a them *(Indicates Kalashnikov.)* is nothin'. But to kill at arm's length requires the deftness of a surgeon and the ferocity of a rabid dog.

(He starts to eat. He indicates the stove.)

[I'm keepin' that on for a special reason.] El Chino says kill without joy. 'Cos the first time you do it it's like sex, you wanna do it, you have to, but you're nervous. Your hands are sweatin'. Your knees are knockin'.

(He stands and puts his beans down.)

And I used to do this, 'cos your lung collapses onto your stomach that's what makes you sick. Y'ad sex? You gotta put your hands underneath your ribcage, bend down, deep breath, straighten up, gun out and shoot the bastard in the back or cock out dependin' on whether it's sex. You gotta remember which it is.

LINGERIE
from <u>Sex and Death</u>
by Diana Amsterdam
New York City - Present - Max (30's)

Max is a womanizing film producer who thinks he has finally fallen in love with a wholesome gal from Georgia. When she refuses to don some sexy lingerie that he has given her, he explodes comically, revealing his unrealistic expectations of their relationship.

MAX: Either you do or you don't. That's all! It's as simple as that. No! I'm not listening to any more arguments. If you love me like you say you do, you put on that lingerie for me. That's all. No! No more arguments. I don't want to hear about your momma and your daddy and God and self respect and rotten commies, we're talking something very real here, very real, loving someone, caring about him enough to want to make him happy. No! I'm not listening. I've tried everything. Reasoning, pleading, cajoling, dressing up like a tart, I've tried it all, I'm not asking you to jump off a cliff, I'm asking you to put on a piece of clothing for me, that's all, if you don't love me enough for that what the hell's gonna happen when something really important comes up! I'll be desperate, you'll be singing the National Anthem, no! No, Sally! There isn't anything more to say! There's the lingerie. There's the champagne. Drink a glass of champagne, put on the lingerie and be a woman to your man, be a woman to your man, take a chance for your man, it's not a lot to ask, it's nothing to ask, no! Sally, if you can't do this much for me, yes, for me, I admit, for me, it's true, for me, okay, for me, what's wrong with that, for me, isn't that love? That we do things for each other? Then I can't stay with you. I'm too vulnerable. I can't trust you to sacrifice for me at all ever, I'm out of here.

18

THE LOMAN FAMILY PICNIC
by Donald Margulies
Coney Island - 1965 - Herbie (40)

Herbie is Stewie's long-suffering father. Constantly struggling to make ends meet, Herbie is on the verge of a breakdown. On the evening following his son's Bar Mitzvah, Herbie explodes with years of pent-up anger and frustration, lashing out at his family and himself with a fury that none suspected he possessed.

HERBIE: *(That did it; he's going berserk.)* YOU THINK I DON'T LOVE YOU?!! YOU THINK I DON'T *LOVE* YOU?!!
(Doris puts her arms protectively around the shaken boys.)
[DORIS: Herbie, shush! The house is shaking!]
HERBIE: *(Jabbing at Stewie.)* I DON'T LOVE YOU?!!
[DORIS: *(Shielding Stewie.)* DON'T HURT HIM!]
HERBIE: LOOK AT YOU WITH YOUR PRECIOUS BOYS! WHAT DO *I* GET, HM?! *(Storms off to bedroom, screaming.)* WHAT DO *I* HAVE! WHAT DO *I* HAVE! *(Doris has her arms around both whimpering boys when Herbie returns carrying a dresser drawer. Now at a terrifying pitch.)* EVERYTHING I HAVE IS HERE IN THIS DRAWER! EVERYTHING I OWN IS RIGHT HERE! I COULD GET THE HELL OUT OF HERE LIKE *THAT!*
[DORIS: Herbie, shhh...]
HERBIE: *(Overlap.)* WHAT DO I *HAVE*?! WHAT'S *MINE*?! THIS MUCH SPACE IN THE CLOSET?! One suit?! You can *keep* the suit; I don't give a damn about that suit; I hate suits; you made me buy that suit.
[DORIS: *(Quietly.)* I thought you needed—]
HERBIE: DONATE IT TO GOODWILL! MAKE BELIEVE I DIED! WEAR IT FOR HALLOWEEN! WHAT DO I HAVE! I HAVE NOTHING! I HAVE SHIT! I HAVE THE TOILET FOR TEN MINUTES IN THE MORNING! I DON'T EVEN HAVE *YOU*!
[DORIS: Herbie...]

19

THE LOMAN FAMILY PICNIC

HERBIE: LOOK AT YOU! LOOK WHO GETS *YOU*!
[DORIS: That's not true—the boys...]
HERBIE: *(Overlap.)* WHAT DO *I* HAVE! I DON'T EVEN
HAVE THE TV! KEEP THE TV! THE HELL WITH THE TV!
I'll buy myself a *new* TV. Top of the line! Color! Yeah, I'll buy
myself a *color*! The boys can have the old one, watch whatever the
hell they want! WHAT DO *I* GET? WHAT DOES *DADDY* GET?
(Shaking the drawer violently.) EVERYTHING IN THE WORLD
THAT'S MINE IS RIGHT HERE IN THIS DRAWER!
EVERYTHING! What do I have? Underwear? This underwear is
shot. Do I buy myself any? Do I buy myself anything? Look at
these socks! Holes! Holes burned through 'em but I wear 'em
anyway, tearing up my feet! My feet are torn up! Do I go to a foot
doctor? Look at all these single, lost socks I hold onto hoping the
other'll show up! Look at this! The hell with them? Garbage!
LOOK AROUND THIS HOUSE! WHAT'S MINE?! NOTHING!
(Rummaging through the drawer.) I got my coin collection! My
silver dollars! What am I? Cufflinks? Tie clips? Skins?
Undershorts with shot elastic? T-shirts with holes under the arms?
THIS IS ME?! THIS IS MY LIFE! THIS DRAWER IS MY
WHOLE LIFE, RIGHT HERE; THIS DRAWER! *(He throws the
drawer down and storms out of the apartment.)*

LOOSE ENDS
by Stuart Hepburn
Glasgow - Present - Spud (40's-50's)

Spud is a former teacher forced into a life of petty crime by his drug addiction. He now lives a meager life in a Glasgow tenement where he barely survives in between jags. Here, he breaks down in front of Callum, a young man whom he has befriended.

SPUD: A doctor? *(Shouts.)* A doctor... I already go to the doctors... *(Defiant.)* Every Wednesday I have to go to the doctors...every fucking Wednesday... *(Defeated.)* Wednesday... *(He calms down.)*
(Silence.)
I get better then I get a jag. *(Shivers.)* It's when I feel cold and it's still warm, before the voices though...I haven't heard them for ages...and I...I talk a lot and use the big words...then I have to get my jag...then it's all right...stops you being depressed...stops you being happy too...sort of...evens you out...flat... *(Smiles.)* But now you could stay 'cause it'll be all right...and the ferries...I could teach you things about the messages...I used to be a teacher...but I got awful cold one day...awful cold, my head was tight... *(Brighter.)* I used to get the kids to call me by my first name... *(Duller.)* that was before the voices... Then when I was cold when my mummy died I just started crying...and they said I had to go...just for a rest, like...to Gartloch...just for a rest...the jag helps you to rest...slows you down...then you don't use the big words...alliteration... *(Laughs.)*
[CALLUM: You were in the hospital?]
SPUD: I'm not a loony, you know, I just needed a rest, I was there for five years...but there was no room left...I go up there to see my friends most days...just for the company like...but, eh... *(Pause. Bright.)* I worked in the gardens...we grew great tomatoes... I go and sit in the gardens...some of my friends aren't there any more... at night I come back here...home...see there wasn't enough room...

21

some of them are in the doss house, or the streets...we had to leave...it would be good if someone could stay here with me though...at home...home...here...the social worker said she would see...said she would see...I wish they'd let us stay but...
(He turns to CALLUM and smiles.)
I get my jag on Wednesday...
(Pause.)
I was just remembering what you said... *(Through tears)* ...about being lonely... I don't want you to go.

A MADHOUSE IN GOA
by Martin Sherman
Greek Islands - 1990 - Oliver (40's)

Oliver is the caretaker of Daniel, a best-selling author whom a
stroke has left unable to communicate. Oliver and Daniel have
spent many years together at Daniel's Greek Island home, and
each depends on the other for daily sustenance. When Oliver
discovers that he has AIDS, he feels that he must leave Daniel
and here tenders his resignation.

OLIVER: Well, look who's up and about. Feeling better, are we?
That's a good boy. Slept well, eh? Four whole days. That's a
record for you. Eyes open to take a little nourishment, then back
shut into never-never land. Four days.
(DANIEL sits down.)
Sitting down, are we, luv? That's good. Do you hear that noise?
Like thunder. In the distance. Spoils the peaceful drone of the
rainfall. Hasn't stopped raining. You didn't miss any sun.
(He looks at DANIEL.)
I guess we were depressed, weren't we? Does your face have more
colour in it? Probably. We like our sleep.
(Pause—he looks away.)
Well—what have you missed? A lot. You've missed a lot.
(Pause.)
Heather's in the hospital. She had a choking fit as soon as Dylan
left. That's when you went to sleep, wasn't it? Yes.
(Pause.)
The cancer has crawled up through her system and is surrounding
her windpipe. Leaning on it, actually. Do you want to hear this?
Do you want to go back to sleep? They think they can reduce it a
bit. They figure she has a few weeks. but you know Heather, she'll
turn weeks into months, if she can. I have a lot of time for Heather.
I'm just afraid the fight may leave her when she hears about Dylan.
(Pause.)
Are you sure you don't want to go back to sleep? I'm not giving

you a needle. Not now.
(Pause.)
Dylan's plane exploded. Everyone dead. A bomb. Hardly got into
the air. Just over the crater. They found some wreckage. On the
cliffs. The explosive device had been placed in a little jewel box.
Pretty clever, eh?
(Pause.)
Are you tired again? What is that sound? I like Dylan. Did you?
It was Aliki, of course. Except her name's not Aliki. It's Maria
something-or-other and she's not Greek, she's Lebanese. Did you
suspect something, you little devil? "Don't sneeze"? What did that
mean? A Palestinian courier had been booked on that flight, that's
supposedly who she was after. He cancelled at the last moment.
They're not sure if she belonged to a Muslim extremist group or
another Palestinian faction or the Israeli secret service. Or the CIA.
Or the KGB. My guess is all of the above. Well, doesn't matter
really, does it? Another gesture for freedom, no matter how you
squeeze it.
(Pause.)
They traced Aliki-or-Maria to Crete. Well, I could have told them
that's where she was. She and Barnaby had taken a hotel room.
They found Barnaby. His throat was cut. Aliki-Maria has
disappeared.
(Pause.)
Thin air.
(Pause.)
Well, you can take some comfort in the knowledge that your book
will never be a musical now. Assuming it upsets you at all.
(Pause.)
I know the world at large would consider you a total mess, but I
rather think you lead a charmed life. I'm not giving you a needle.
What is that noise?
(Pause.)
I'm leaving you. I've placed an advertisement in the *Herald-Tribune*

for a replacement. I'll find you someone very convivial. It seems that I myself am on a sinking ship. I'm waving goodbye as well. Do you understand? I found a lesion on my arm. I had the necessary tests. I have AIDS. I suppose it can be classified as ironic. The last time I was with someone was five years ago. And only for a minute. Well—so it goes.
(Pause.)
It hasn't registered yet, really. I'm numb. I'm not even angry or sad. Just numb. Funny, that.
(Pause.)
But I am quite sure of one thing and that's that I'm not ending my days with you.
(Pause.)
I used to work in a clinic. Didn't get paid well. But it meant something. It helped. I have healing gifts. Don't I, luv? I think I've been wasting them on you. But right now, with this odd numbness, everything seems wasted.
(Pause.)
I don't hate you. Don't think that. But if you have gifts, you should use them, shouldn't you? It's a way of facing the madness and shouting 'stop'. You, of course, can't even say 'stop'. If you tried, it would come out as ice-cream.
(Pause.)
So you've missed a lot. It pays to stay awake these days.
(Pause.)
What stories are you writing in your head? What faces do you see? Do the heavens dance? Does a star fall on Albania? Do you feel the cool breeze from the Levant? Does the breeze comfort you? Do you know at last what it means?

THE MAN WHO LOST AMERICA
by Michael Burrell
Saratoga, NY - 1777 - General Burgoyne (40's-50's)

At the close of the American Revolutionary War, General
Burgoyne hides himself away while awaiting an opportunity to
return to England. Defeated and bitter, the General surveys his
hiding place and wonders what to say to his friends when he
returns home.

OFFICER: It's not Drury Lane but it'll do. Indeed, I have seen
actors in worse dressing-rooms. Perhaps this is a taste of the future.
(He places the lantern where it sheds a little more light.)
We negotiated with them as gentlemen. And as gentlemen we
concluded an agreement. Then they broke it. Like gentlemen.
They're the official enemy so it was on the cards. But what do you
say to your official friends, who are always so much more vicious?
Especially the ones you were at school with. God knows. I'll have
to think of something.
*(He goes to the blanket over the window and releases it. A shaft of
light breaks through, making the room much more visible though
hardly bright.)*
The weather could be English: cold, motionless and not too bright.
So. What to say, how to carry it off? It'll be the nail or the nose-
gay for my reputation. Bribery would probably work best, at least
with my friends. Can't afford that. Shipwreck on the way home?
It would be a solution, in every sense. With some appeal, Charlotte,
you know that. But it lacks bottom and it wouldn't answer. Which
leaves—a little wit, a little intelligence, a sharp memory and the
truth. Tell 'em the truth, all of it. Yes, that should bring about the
second great disaster of my career. Friends at home are so
fastidious. Everything must be filtered, whether it's sunlight or
mulled wine or uncomfortable facts, passed through a sieve so that
any grossness may be purged. Truth is so often so inconvenient.
(He blows out the lantern.)
It's the wits, then, and as much courage as I can muster. And deep
preparation as always, so I shan't be taken by surprise.

MINNA AND THE SPACE PEOPLE
from <u>Family Life</u>
by Wendy Hammond
A mental hospital - Present - Brett (30's)

Brett visits his sister, Minna, in a mental hospital. Minna is
pregnant and claims that benevolent space people have given her
the child that will eventually save the world from nuclear war.
Here, Brett pleads with Minna to have an abortion.

BRETT: YOU   BELIEVE   IN   SPACE   PEOPLE!   THAT'S
CRAZY!!!!
[MINNA: *(Deep breath)* You mean you're not going to help me?]
[BRETT: No.]
[MINNA: You won't help save the savior of the world?]
[BRETT: No.]
[MINNA: What if Jesus had been an abortion? Think of that.]
[BRETT: Jesus' mother didn't live in a nuthouse.]
*(Beside herself, MINNA kicks a chair, then plops down into it, facing
away from BRETT.)*
BRETT: Minna, someday, if you do everything the doctors tell you,
maybe you'll get out of here. And then you'll find a job and a
husband and then you can start a family, a normal family. Isn't that
what you really want? Isn't that the way you really want it?
(MINNA doesn't respond.) Minna, come on. Talk to me, OK?
(MINNA doesn't respond.) I just think it'll be easier to have this
abortion now than to give the baby away later. *(MINNA doesn't
respond.)* You know I'm right. I know you know I'm right.
(MINNA doesn't respond.) Minna, we gotta talk about this. We're
not going to get anywhere if we don't start talking. *(MINNA doesn't
respond. BRETT picks up the Christmas present and drops it in
MINNA's lap.)* The least you could do is open your Christmas
present.
*(MINNA rips the bow and paper off, opens the box, and pulls out a
scarf and a glass fish. She reaches into her bra and takes out a
lighter.)*

MINNA AND THE SPACE PEOPLE

[BRETT: Where did you get that? You're not supposed to have that! *(MINNA sets the scarf on fire.)* MINNA!]

(BRETT lunges for the scarf, throws it on the ground, and stomps the fire out. Meanwhile MINNA has picked up the fish and calmly placed it on the floor. She stomps on the fish, smashing it into tiny pieces of glass.)

BRETT: MINNA MINNA! STOP IT STOP IT! *(But the glass fish is destroyed. BRETT crosses to the glass bits and begins picking them up. MINNA stands, watching him. BRETT is blinking back tears.)* I spent three lunch hours shopping for this. Three! I could have been clearing my desk. I could have been making phone calls or seeing clients or dictating reports, but no, I was searching and searching for the exact perfect replica of the little glass fish you had when we were kids. And now you've smashed it to bits. Three hours wasted. I work 'til nine every night, do you have any idea what that's like? I get home at ten, eat, do the dishes, take the garbage out, go to bed, then get up at 5:30 the next morning and start the whole thing again! I ask Rita to help with the garbage but...well, things can get tense in a marriage... And now you want to have a baby and I don't care WHAT you say I just know I'M the one who's going to end up taking care of you AND your baby and Rita's not going to like that at ALL, not at ALL! And when Rita doesn't like things...well I don't want to talk about Rita. Don't move. You'll cut yourself.

MISS EVERS' BOYS
by David Feldshuh
Tuskegee, Alabama - 1932-1972 - Caleb (30-40)

Caleb and three of his friends have been diagnosed with syphilis and are participating in a government funded project to study the effects of the disease on the Black male. Unknown to the patients, they are not being treated for the disease so that the government can study its unchecked effects. Here, Caleb is about to receive a spinal tap, and his fear of the procedure reminds him of a terrible day in his youth.

CALEB: You know I was raised Baptist and I'm thinking that when you're raised Baptist you got a better chance of being a "talking man" 'cause if you got a good preacher preaching at you each week, you get a feeling for it.
[EVERS: That's what you had?]
CALEB: [Yes, ma'am. Every week.] Reverend Banks he was a fine preacher. As far back as I can remember back, I can remember his preaching. When I was six years old a big lightning storm touched down by the church. The church members said that lightning was just plain jealous of the voice of Reverend Banks. Well, an old oak tree was cut down by that lightning and fell on the outhouse behind the church. The next Sunday I climbed up on that oak tree and started taking off on the Reverend to the other children. "Raise out of hell"; "Keep you eyes on the Lord"; then I warmed up, didn't care what I was saying anymore: "This here tree has brushed this here outhouse 'cause it smelled; smelled; smelled so bad"... I'm goin' on like that in the biggest, deepest voice a six-year-old can put on and the Reverend hear me, my mother hear me, the whole choir that's practicing just inside the church while we kids is playing outside, they hear me too. And I was lashed for the wages of sin. This back shot can't hurt worse than that day. After that, every time we were alone, all those children would be yelling at me, "Caleb, Caleb, do the Reverend. Do the Reverend." Now I "do the Reverend" for the fun of it.

29

MISS EVERS' BOYS
by David Feldshuh
Tuskegee, Alabama - 1932-1972 - Dr. Brodus (40-50)

Dr. Brodus is the Black doctor working in conjuction with the
government in the syphilis study. When confronted by the
dedicated nurse who has been working with the infected men and
demands that they be given treatment for the disease, Brodus
responds by reminding her that they now have an opportunity to
force the medical community to acknowledge physiological
equality between the races.

BRODUS *(After a moment)*: I once did two autopsies at the same
time. On two patients, both in their thirties. On two tables. Laid
out next to each other. I took out the hearts and put them on a scale
and weighted them both. Together. Then I went about some other
business. When I came back I realized I hadn't tagged those hearts.
I didn't know which one came from which table. Now that was
more than embarrassing. You see there was a white man laid out on
one table and a colored man on the other. Now if I put the white
heart in the colored patient... Or the colored heart in the white
patient... So I looked at those hearts for a long time. I held them
both up in my hands, examining them. For the longest time... Then
I closed my eyes and put a heart in each body and sewed them up.
As simple as that. *(Pause.)* Nurse Evers, you and I got a chance to
do something special right now. We got a chance to push people to
see things in a way they've never seen them before. Push them to
see past the hate, past the idea of difference... Isn't that what we've
got to do?

MY CHILDREN! MY AFRICA!
by Athol Fugard
Camdeboo, South Africa - 1985 - Mr. M (40's)

Anela Myalata teaches school in a black township in South Africa. Known as "Mr. M" to his students, Anela has long been an inspiration to the young minds which he helps to guide through the treacherous world of apartheit. When he discovers that his finest students have organized an illegal political action committee, he reports those who have influenced them to the police. Here, he defends his actions to young Thami, his favorite student.

MR. M: *(HE makes his confession simply and truthfully.)* That's right, Thami. I am guilty. I did go to the police. I sat down in Captain Lategan's office and told him I felt it was my duty to report the presence in our community of strangers from the north. I told him that I had reason to believe that they were behind the present unrest. I gave the Captain names and addresses. He thanked me and offered me money for the information, which I refused.

(Pause.) Why do you look at me like that? Isn't that what you expected from me?... A government stooge, a sell-out, an arse-licker? Isn't that what you were all secretly hoping I would do...so that you could be proved right? *(Appalled.)* Is that why I did it? Out of spite? Can a man destroy himself, his life for a reason as petty as that?

I sat here before going to the police station saying to myself that it was my duty, to my conscience, to you, to the whole community to do whatever I could to put an end to this madness of boycotts and arson, mob violence and lawlessness...and maybe that is true...but only maybe...because, Thami, the truth is that I was so lonely! You had deserted me. I was so jealous of those who had taken you away. *Now*, I've *really* lost you, haven't I? Yes. I can see it in your eyes. You'll never forgive me for doing that, will you?

You know, Thami, I'd sell my soul to have you all back behind your desks for one last lesson. Yes. If the devil thought it was worth having and offered me that in exchange...one lesson! He

31

MY CHILDREN! MY AFRICA!

could have my soul. So then it's all over! Because this... *(The classroom.)* ...is all there was for me. This was my home, my life, my one and only ambition...to be a good teacher! *(His dictionary.)* Anela Myalata, twenty years old, from Cookhouse, wanted to be that the way your friends wanted to be big soccer stars playing for Kaizer Chiefs! That ambition goes back to when he was just a skinny little ten-year-old pissing on a small grey bush at the top of the Wapadsberg Pass.

We were on our way to a rugby match at Somerset East. The lorry stopped at the top of the mountain so that we could stretch our legs and relieve ourselves. It was a hard ride on the back of that lorry. The road hadn't been tarred yet. So there I was, ten years old and sighing with relief as I aimed for the little bush. It was a hot day. The sun right over our heads...not a cloud in the vast blue sky. I looked out...it's very high up there at the top of the pass... and there it was, stretching away from the foot of the mountain, the great pan of the Karoo...stretching away forever, it seemed, into the purple haze and heat of the horizon. Something grabbed my heart at that moment, my soul, and squeezed it until there were tears in my eyes. I had never seen anything so big, so beautiful in all my life. I went to the teacher who was with us and asked him: "Teacher, where will I come to if I start walking that way"...and I pointed. He laughed. "Little man," he said, "that way is north. If you start walking that way and just keep on walking, and your legs don't give in, you will see all of Africa! Yes, Africa, little man! You will see the great rivers of the continent: the Vaal, the Zambesi, the Limpopo, the Congo and then the mighty Nile. You will see the mountains: the Drakensberg, Kilimanjaro, Kenya and the Ruwenzori. And you will meet all our brothers: the little Pygmies of the forests, the proud Masai, the Watusi...tallest of the tall and the Kikuyu standing on one leg like herons in a pond waiting for a frog." "Has teacher seen all that?" I asked. "No," he said. "Then how does teacher know it's there?" "Because it is all in the books and I have read the books and if you work hard in school, little man, you can do the same without worrying about your legs giving in."

MY CHILDREN! MY AFRICA!

He was right, Thami. *I* have seen it. It is all there in the books just as he said it was and I have made it mine. I can stand on the banks of all those great rivers, look up at the majesty of all those mountains, whenever I want to. It is a journey I have made many times. Whenever my spirit was low and I sat alone in my room, I said to myself: Walk, Anela! Walk!...and I imagined myself at the foot of the Wapadsberg setting off for that horizon that called me that day forty years ago. It always worked! When I left that little room, I walked back into the world a proud man, because I was an African and all the splendor was my birthright.

(Pause.) I don't want to make that journey again, Thami. There is someone waiting for me now at the end of it who has made a mockery of all my visions of splendor. He has in his arms my real birthright. I saw him on the television in the Reverend Mbop's lounge. An Ethiopian tribesman, and he was carrying the body of a little child that had died of hunger in the famine...a small bundle carelessly wrapped in a few rags. I couldn't tell how old the man was. The lines of despair and starvation on his face made him look as old as Africa itself.

He held that little bundle very lightly as he shuffled along to a mass grave, and when he reached it, he didn't have the strength to kneel and lay it down gently... He just opened his arms and let it fall. I was very upset when the program ended. Nobody had thought to tell us his name and whether he was the child's father, or grandfather, or uncle. And the same for the baby! Didn't it have a name? How dare you show me one of our children being thrown away and not tell me its name! I demand to know who is in that bundle!

(Pause.) Not knowing their names doesn't matter anymore. They are more than just themselves. The tribesmen and dead child do duty for all of us, Thami. Every African soul is either carrying that bundle or in it.

What is wrong with this world that it wants to waste you all like that...my children...my Africa! *(Holding out a hand as if he wanted to touch Thami's face.)* My beautiful and proud young Africa!

SEIZE THE FIRE
by Tom Paulin
Ancient Greece - Prometheus (20-30)

Prometheus rages against Zeus for his imprisonment and begs
for death so that he may at least become one of the people that
he so dearly loves.

PROMETHEUS: Holy Mother, Themis, Earth,
it must all break
here in this wet yard
at the world's end
where they design pain
in secret for me
and cross my name—
my whole nature out—
by writing REBEL
then mocking me for what I'm not.
Men, women, tiny kids,
every juicy little life—
Zeus wanted crush them.
I heard their stittering
frantic cries,
cries like pebbles bouncing
on a stone floor,
and my conviction
was simple and complete.
That's why I stole
that restless, bursting,
tight germ of fire,
and chucked its flames
like a splatter of raw paint
against his state.
They seized the running trails
and ran with them,
every mind fizzing like resin—

SEIZE THE FIRE

racing, dancing, leaping free,
jumping up into the sky,
and nudging deep
into the ocean's bottom.
Every mind was a splinter
of sharp, pure fire
that needled him
and made him rock
uneasy on his throne.
See Zeus, shaken
as these new lights burn
and melt his walls.
Let Prometheus go out
and become one
with the democratic light!

THE WIDOW'S BLIND DATE
by Israel Horovitz
Massachusetts - Present - Archie (30's)

Archie is a brutish sort of fellow who works the baler in his uncle's factory. When Margy, the woman whom he has loved since the second grade, returns to town to visit her dying brother, Archie is surprised and pleased when she invites him out to dinner. She meets him at the factory, and he attempts to entertain her with a story of his childhood in the factory.

ARCHIE: When I was a little guy, I used to work here every Saturday. I got two bucks, which was a big deal then...wicked big. *(Smiles.)* Used ta be maybe seven, eight winos used ta work here weekends...for my Uncle Max...before Spike the Loon worked with us... I was just a kid. *(Pauses; lost in a memory.)* "Lum" is what we called the big one. His name was Alfred, I think... Some people called him Allie. Most of us called him "Lumbago" on accounta he had it. For short, we called him "Lum." Dumbest, meanest son-of-a-bitch ten towns around, and that's a fact. *(Pauses.)* My particular specialty was to climb into the baler, counta I was a kid and little and all, and push the newspapers tight into the corners. A good bale has sharp edges. The only thing was, getting inside the press spooked me. Gave me the willies... *(Pauses.)* Lum always used to threaten me when I was in here. He used ta say he'd pull the top over me when I was inside. Then he'd say they'd press me in with the overissues and sell me in the bale and I'd get driven up to Fitchburg, to Felulah's Mill, and I'd get dumped into the acid bath with the overissues and come out ta the wet press up there, rolled into fine paper for stationery... *(Pauses.)* The miserable son-of-a-bitch! Tellin' that to a kid, huh? He grabbed me in a headlock one Saturday, right here on this spot. Lum. No warning at all. He just grabbed me. I figured I was a dead kid, ya know. I mean, I was eleven and he was forty. The odds weren't exactly on *me*, ya know what I mean? But, I took a major shot and I whipped him around backwards. *(He looks at George, who averts his eyes.)* I ran

36

myself forward as fast as I could, whipping him around so hard, it was like his face exploded. It looked ta' me like his head was half opened up. He landed on the stack, and just lay there, blood oozing out of him, staining the papers. *(Pauses.)* I figured I'd killed him. *(Pauses.)* Winos grumblin', lookin' this way and that. ...They started fadin' outta the shop...the winos. *(Pauses.)* I was scared shit. Just me alone and the body: Lum. *(Pauses.)* I figured the cops would give me the electric chair...or worse; hangin'... *(Pauses.)* I was scared shit. *(Pauses.)* I figured the only way was to get rid of the body, hide him. The winos wouldn't talk. Nobody'd miss him, anyway, right? *(Pauses.)* I started coverin' him up with newspaper, but his blood kept staining through. So, I started draggin' him over to the baler...to throw him in. I was only eleven, Marg. Can you get the picture? *(Archie moves to baler to better illustrate his story. George will soon move in closer to Margy and this time, Archie will register jealously. Without a break in story-telling, Archie will shove Geroge aside and complete his story.)* Me, eleven, draggin' this forty-year-old-drunken corpse by the arm to the press here... *(Pause.)* This very very one... *(Slaps baler, pauses, smiles.)* You'll never guess what happened Marg. You'll never in a million years guess what happened, Marg. You'll never in a million years guess... *(Laughs.)* Gave me bad dreams for about eighteen years... *(Pauses.)* Lum got up. I swear to God. He opens his eyes...blinks a bunch a'times...and then...then... *(He laughs.)* Lum gets up, as though from the dead. The cut wasn't all that deep, just bleedin' wicked. He must'a been out as much from the wine as from the hitting the baler. Blood dripping all down him... He comes at me. *(Pauses.)* I figured he was gonna kill me, Margy. Get even. He didn't. He shook his head a couple of times...moves to his chino Eisenhower jacket, and he goes away. No pay. No finishin' the day. No attempt whatsoever to do damage to me. *(Pauses.)* That was a big day in the life of this little Arnold "Billy-Goat" Crisp. I can tell you that. *(Pauses.)* Gaining respect is what life is all about.

THE WIDOW'S BLIND DATE
by Israel Horovitz
Massachusetts - Present - George (30's)

George is an illiterate womanizer helping out his friend, Archie,
in the baling press room at a wastepaper factory. When the two
men are visited by Margy, a childhood friend, George becomes
irritated by her refined mannerisms. He lashes out at her, his
jealously of her attention to Archie showing.

GEORGE: I don't like this. *(Pauses.)* I'd like to point out to you,
Archie, that this Margy Palumbo is tryin'...and succeedin'...in
making goddam fools...idiots!...out ta the rotten two of us.
[MARGY: Archie, I'm not doing that.]
GEORGE: You think Archie Crisp is just some jerk kid you can
fuck over, huh? Fuck him over for a laugh and then scoot, right out
and spend the next fifteen/twenty years tellin' you high-fallootin'
friends about this local, see?... This *local*...this townie asshole,
Archie Crisp...and how he came on to her. Still likin' her and all,
after all those years since the second grade. *(Imitates Margy talking
to a cultured friend.)* This Archie Crisp, you see, is what you'd call
a really steady boyfriend... How steady? Second grade right up till
age thirty-five/forty... How's *that* for steady, huh? Those locals
stick like glue, huh? Not much goin' in those locals' lives, huh?...
Couple of farmers, 'ceptin' they got no *farms! (He bales furiously.)*
She's insulting us, Archie! That's it—she's putting us down!
[ARCHIE: Shut it up, Geroge, huh? Huh? Huhhh? You got the
brains of a cruller. *(Tosses a bundle into baler.)* Leave me out of
this. I'm just doing my work.]
GEORGE: You're her supper date, right? I mean she called you,
not me?... I'm just being friendly and all...not comin' on or causin'
trouble or nothin'...just bein' friendly and all...for old time's sake...
(Pauses.) And for the sake of our old buddy, Swede...who's kicking
off... *(Archie looks at George.)* ...out of memory for the Moose...
and her former junior high steady, our own Spike and Loon...dearly
departed...and account a she's got kids, Raymond, et cetera, and her

38

THE WIDOW'S BLIND DATE

bein' unhappy and all...mentally fuckin' *depressed!* *(George is moving toward Margy now.)* We behaved respectably with you on account of all those things, Margy, and what I hear is that you can't stop laughin' at us and insultin' us and playing it smart...playin' it smart... *(He lifts bundle up over her head, menacingly.)* I've got muscle now, Margy. That's one change from the old days, right? Me, rolley-polley and all... That's one change you might a noticed, huh? Geroge Ferguson ain't rolley-polley now! Opposite: Geroge Ferguson is a well developed man... He's strong... He can lift... He's got muscle... Uh huh. *(He throws bundle at Archie.)* You workin' or you watchin', huh? If you want a bale wired and out and ready for your fat uncle at four o'clock, you got ta move on it, same as me... *(To Margy.)* I personally never held with the idea that women are weak and along for a free ride. *(He throws a bundle to her.)* Up and into the baler. MOVE! *(Margy catches bundle and throws it at the baler's front door, screaming primal scream.)* I do not like the attitude you've got right now! I think your pronouns are fucked up, too! I can't follow your ante-fuckin'-cedents!
[ARCHIE: Cool down, George. You're hot...]
GEORGE: *I'm hot, alright... I'm hot.* Why not, huh? How'm I gonna stay cool with Miss Margy Palumbo blowin' in my ear like she does, huh? *(Turns to Margy, then to Archie.)* This pisses me off. *This just pisses me off.* *(Grabs two bundles, throws them into the baler.)* This just pisses me off! *(To Margy.)* What you're after here is trouble between me and Archie. That's the way I got it pegged. You get your kicks outta' causin' us to be fightin' and crap with each other. That's the way I got it pegged... *(To Archie.)* And I got a good eye. I got a good eye. *(To Margy.)* I don't like the way you call me and Archie here dumb or stupid for not gettin' our pictures in the *Item* the way you do... *(Displays newspaper photo.)* What's this anway, huh? Does this mean that if anything... you know...happened to you, that a lot of people would come snoopin' around on accounta' you're famous, so's they noticed you were missing kinda' thing?

THE WIDOW'S BLIND DATE

[MARGY: My children...Raymond and Rosie...they'd miss me...
They'd "come snoopin'"...]
GEORGE: I don't like you using your sex on us the way you do...
to split us up...me and my best friend, Archie...

THE BOYS OF WINTER
by John Pielmeier
Viet Nam - December, 1968 - Monsoon (18)

When Bonney, an American GI in Viet Nam, commits a war crime, the men of his unit are questioned about his state of mind. Here, Monsoon, a racist young southerner, reveals his new insight into ethnic differences gained on the battlefield.

MONSOON: I mean when I was a kid, sir, it was nigger this nigger that my Daddy braggin about how he strung up some darkey just for *lookin* at a white woman I mean I got my Klan membership and everything and lo and behold I'm over here cryin my eyes out and this goddamn black man's offerin me his hanky! I couldn't fuckin believe it! But that's the secret, sir, I mean the battlefield's the only one hundred percent pure goddamn democracy we'll ever know I mean them bullets they got *no* prejudice. So here I am holed up with this brother and we're cryin together and shittin together and sleepin so close I could feel his breath—I woke up one night and I saw the moon dancin on his skin, this part in the throat right here with his heart beatin against it, and I swore if Charlie did anything to that dude I'd tear the motherfucker's head off. That's the reason for most of the shit, sir, your buddy trusts you with his life, some gook pops him in the head, the next coupla dinks you see you're gonna send to fuckin Buddha, no questions asked, cause they ain't worth one beat of his heart against this place in the throat.

And that's why, sir. Why three days after he got back Bonney walked into that ville and wasted seven gooks, no questions asked. One for each of us, sir, himself included.

THE BOYS OF WINTER
by John Pielmeier
Viet Nam - December, 1968 - Doc (20)

Here, the unusually insightful Doc points the finger of blame where it truly belongs.

DOC: Funny thing about this war, sir, it got us doin shit we'da never dreamed possible. I hear about this My Lai and now the shit that Bonney pulled and I don't condone it, sir, but we all did it. We all have little My Lai's in the corners of our souls, you as well as me, and this war just pointed em out a little more clearly. I mean you gun down some old women and a bunch of kids there's not much more you can learn about yourself, know what I mean? You stand there wonderin how the hell Bonney coulda done it and I just thank my lucky stars it wasn't me.

So don't blame *him*, sir. You're the ones taught us how to kill. I mean if this country gonna fight a war you gotta take responsibilities for the casualties of that war. You don't bring em to trial. You don't ignore em when they ask for help. You don't not celeberate what they tried to do for their country. You understand what I'm sayin? Responsibility has got to be taken! You betrayed us, sir, you and Kennedy and Johnson, General Westmoreland, John Wayne, *(flinging the blood)* you lied to us, you're a bunch of fuckin old men, you were jealous cause we were too goddam young!

It's you. *You're* the ones shoulda been thrown into a ditch and shot. Sir.
(He salutes. MONSOON begins screaming.)

THE BOYS OF WINTER
by John Pielmeier
Viet Nam - December, 1968 - L.B. (18)

The tragic horror of Viet Nam is expressed in the following painful observations which eloquently link sex and death.

L.B.: Sex and death!
(Silence. A white light hits him.)
Sex and death. You wanna know the truth, sir, I got it all figured out.

See here I am two months in-country and all of a once I'm caught in this firefight with my pants down takin a shit, see, and this brother starts crawlin up to me with his stomach in his hands—hold on, sir, I got a point to make here I mean you wanna get to the bottom of this, right?—so I kinda tuck this brother back together and I'm lyin there waitin for the duster with my hand up to my wrist inside him and my pants down around my ankles and I'm thinkin, Shit, man, I ain't ever been this intimate with Bernice. And all of a once, sir, I start to kinda like it, you know what I mean? I mean here I am ain't had a woman for months about ready to fuck this guy in the stomach and all of a once I realize that that's what this war's all about. Fuckin and dyin, fuckin and dyin, got so you can't tell the difference, I mean best fucks I ever had was the Quang Tri whores cause they had that look in their eye you know? I mean we were intercoursin the whole country, sir, let's face it. Save em from Communism, bullshit, America just want a little pussy. And the Marines in the field, man, they're ashamed cause they're rapin twelve-year-old girls, humpin grandmothers, and it's so terrible, man, you can't drag youself away. The tracers in the night, I never seen anything so beautiful, napalm, white phosphorous, gorgeous, baby. And all of a once it got so you just as soon shoot em instead of fuck em. Every time you seen a body your heart took a leap cause it wasn't you, man, that was the mind-fuck of it all, you were still *alive*.

43

THE COCKTAIL HOUR
by A.R. Gurney
Upstate New York - 1970's - Bradley (70's)

As the family gathers for a cocktail hour before dinner, Bradley, the patriarch of the WASP-ish clan, laments the fact that no one drinks anymore.

BRADLEY: *(Now pouring his own scotch and water very carefully.)* Of course, nobody drinks much these days. At least not with any relish. Marv Watson down at the club is now completely on the wagon. You sit down beside him at the big table, and what's he drinking? Orange juice. I said, "Am I confused about the time, Marv? Are we having breakfast?" Of course the poor thing can't hear, so it doesn't make any difference. But you go to parties these days and even the young people aren't drinking. I saw young Kathy Bickford at the Shoemaker wedding. Standing on the sidelines, looking very morose indeed. I went up to her and said, "What's that strange concoction you've got in your hand, Kathy?" She said, "Lemon Squirt." I said, "What?" She said, "Sugar-free, noncarbonated Lemon Squirt." So I said, "Now, Kathy, you listen to me. You're young and attractive, and you should be drinking champagne. You should be downing a good glass of French champagne, one, two, three, and then you should be out there on that dance floor, kicking up your heels with every usher in sight. And after you've done that, you should come right back here, and dance with me!" Of course, she walked away. *(He finishes making his drink.)* They all walk away these days. I suppose I'm becoming a tiresome old fool.

DARKSIDE
by Ken Jones
A bar - 1973 - Gerald R. "Gunner" Smith (30-40)
Here, an experienced astronaut describes taking off in a Saturn
V rocket to a couple of rookies. As he speaks, we can see his
love for his work.

GUNNER: You're lying on your back. Looking up at your feet.
After about an hour of holding for some small problem, you begin
to lose your sense of direction. Then Mission Control starts to call
out the last ten. You feel the beast breathing. You can hear it
groaning beneath you. You begin to tremble ever so gently growing
slowly into a quake. A pounding of your whole being. But you're
still not moving!

[BILL: Jesus.]

GUNNER: You look out the windows, and through the flames, way
in the distance, you can see the birds flying away. Those poor birds
trying to escape the heat.

[ED: 160 million horse power! Holy shit!]

GUNNER: But then, out of an ocean of fire, you start to climb.
But it's not like the Atlas rockets. It's slow. Dead slow. Inches.
Feet. Yards. Miles! Now you're moving! 9,300 feet per second!
In three minutes you're seventy miles away from the launch tower.
You've got 4 G's pushing you back into your seat.

[BILL: Is it loud?]

GUNNER: It sounds like the heavens cracking. It's Genesis and
Armaggedon all rolled into one. Pretty soon the sound can't even
keep up. And all of a sudden, you come flying out of your chair,
smashing into your harness, almost crashing into your instrument
panel. Your whole system freezes up. You're scared to move until
Houston reminds you that you've just lost your first stage. And now
there is the silence. The silence that you pray will be shattered by
the sound of the second stage lighting up. You wait. Listening.
Hoping. And—boom! The beast comes back to life with a
vengeance and rams you right in the seat of your pants. You sink
deeper and deeper into your chair. Like you're going to melt right
into it. And then, you punch through. You're in space. You're
finally, free.

DEALING WITH CLAIR
by Martin Crimp
London - Present - James (50's)

The mysterious James has made a cash offer on a house being shown by Clair. James appears to be attracted to the young realtor and here reveals uncanny insight into her life.

JAMES: I'll tell you something. And of course I may be completely wrong. But I'm pretty certain you have one of those beds, don't you, that folds up into a sofa. Is that right? Look, I'm sorry, I'm not embarrassing you am I? All I mean is, is it begins as a sofa. You spend the evening sitting on it, most probably on your own. Then at a certain time, and although the time is utterly up to you, it's probably always the same time near enough, you get off the sofa, and you unfold it and rearrange it in a special way which once seemed rather complicated but now comes to you as second nature, and you get ready for bed and you get into it. Please stop me if I'm wrong. And in the morning you are woken by the alarm—if not by the trains—and you get up, and you get ready for work. But before you go out, you turn the bed back into a sofa again. Except on those days—and this is the nub—except on those days when you're late for work perhaps, or you simply can't face it, you simply can't face folding the bloody thing up. So you leave it. But the moment you get home in the evening you take one look at it, you take one look at it and you regret having left it like that. Unmade like that. Bitterly. Because immediately there is a dilemma. I don't think it's too much to speak of a dilemma, do you. And the last thing any of us wants is a dilemma, particularly in the evenings. Because either you turn your bed back into a sofa, knowing that in a few hours you'll have to turn your sofa into a bed again. Or of course you leave it. The disadvantage in this case being that desolate feeling that nothing in the room has really happened to distinguish between morning, evening, and night.

46

EASTERN STANDARD
by Richard Greenberg
Fire Island - Present - Peter (20's-30)

A successful television executive, Peter has been diagnosed as being HIV positive. He instinctively retreats from reality by joining his sister and her lover, Stephen, at Stephen's summer house on Fire Island. Here, Peter offers Stephen a glimpse into the lifestyle that brought about his tragic end.

PETER: That's how it was, entering a room... Lovers everywhere. People you'd had, people you might soon have. Oh God, and the way you stared and the way you were stared at. You could fall in love with anything—a jawline, a chin—because it didn't have to last beyond the half-hour. And everything was understood; no negotiations that made you lose your appetite for the prize. You'd see someone, you'd find him early; and you didn't think—is he going to like me, is he smart, will we have anything to talk about? No, you thought: there's my evening. And the glitter in his eyes, taking you in as if you were a newly-discovered continent. And it might last an hour, or sometimes a day, or some amazing times a month, but it never got stale, because the minute you felt yourself start to become boring, you'd just click away—scarcely even saying goodbye. And never—never—any regret, because there was always someone else who'd fall in love with you a few minutes away.

A GIRL'S GUIDE TO CHAOS
by Cynthia Heimel
New York City - Present - Jake (20-30)

Here, Jake speaks to the audience of his experience with
relationships and offers insight into the sometimes befuddling
realm of romance in the 1980's.

JAKE: Now I was monogamous. Faithful old Jake. Cynthia was
more than enough for me to handle. We lived together for three
years. I think I scared her away. I came on too strong. I knew
what I wanted, and I took it. Tried to take it. You know what she
used to love? Going to the supermarkets at three in the morning.
She was always looking for the plums with the red meat inside them.
She'd get this excited look in her eye as she stuck her thumbnail into
each plum.

Women! There's someone else I have my eye on now. It's a
little complicated. Don't even ask. And you know, I'm trying to do
it just right. I don't call every day. I call maybe every fourth day.
And I try for nonchalance. *(WHISTLES, TWIDDLES FINGER.)* So,
like, wanna go to a movie maybe?

I've gotten nowhere. She doesn't even know I exist. I think.
I don't know. I'm confused.

Here's my theory: You live in New York of all places, in 1988
of all times, and you can't help it, you're totally self-involved.

We all not only think we're the center of the universe and about
to become famous in a second, but we're completely self-conscious.
Like me being nonchalant. Like me searching my soul for the
proper place to take her for cappuccino to make a good impression.
Is Zabar's too yuppie? Is Lanciani too bright? I edit what I say—I
remember in the sixties when you could just say, "Come here,
woman," and then in the seventies you just got a look in your eye
like your puppy died and said, "I know I shouldn't be telling you
this, but I cry sometimes, late at night." Now I don't know. So I
just say what comes into my mind. That doesn't work either.

I mean, what's the big deal? Why is searching for a mate

suddenly on the scale of the Crusades? Why can't we just be with someone, say, "Okay, I have fun with you, I like to sleep with you, you're the one for me, I'm going to stop looking now."

Hah! Wake me when we get things figured out.

HAPGOOD
by Tom Stoppard
Indoor shooting range - Present - Kerner (40's)

Kerner is a Russian physicist turned double agent in his new life
in the west. The ever-cryptic Kerner here discusses Einstein and
God with Mrs. Hapgood, a senior level British spy.

KERNER: It upset Einstein very much, you know, all that damned
quantum jumping, it spoiled his idea of God, which I tell you frankly
is the only idea of Einstein's I never understood. He believed in the
same God as Newton, causality, nothing without reason, but now
one thing led to another until causality was dead. Quantum
mechanics made everything finally random, things can go this way
or that way, the mathematics deny certainty, they reveal only
probability and chance, and Einstein couldn't believe in a God who
threw dice. He should have come to me, I would have told him,
'Listen, Albert, He threw *you*—look around, He never stops.' What
is a hamster, by the way? No, tell me in a minute, I want to tell
you something first. There is a straight ladder from the atom to the
grain of sand, and the only real mystery in physics is the missing
rung. Below it, particle physics; above it, classical physics; but in
between, metaphysics. All the mystery in life turns out to be this
same mystery, the join between things which are distinct and yet
continuous, body and mind, free will and fate, living cells and life
itself; the moment before the foetus. Who needed God when
everything worked like billiard balls? *(He laughs quietly to himself.)*
The man who took the certainty out of Newton was Einstein. *Da!*
He supplied the dice. If there's no God it's a terrible waste of a
good joke. What were you going to say?

LLOYD'S PRAYER
by Kevin Kling
Small town in mid-America - Present - Lloyd (30-50)

When Lloyd is released from prison, he immediately embarks
upon a career as an evangelist. Here, the wiley con-artist
welcomes unsuspecting victims to "Lloyd's Holy World."

LLOYD: Hello, brothers and sisters, and welcome to Lloyd's Holy
World, the place for all your spiritual needs. Be it plastic, wood or
paper we've got it at Lloyd's. You know, friends, I've shopped
some of the other spiritual outlet stores and one look at those prices
and I wept. Why, I could sooner fit through the eye of a camel than
afford. We've got calendars here... Daily memos, ashtrays...a
slightly used beast boy cage, we've got it all. And don't forget to
bring the kids, because for every child under sixteen we have a free
salvation mystery ring. See, they magically change colors and reveal
hidden secrets about your soul. Nice, huh? And get a load of this...
The surprise faith grab-bag barrel. I won't tell you what's in here
but I do give my personal guarantee that each and every item is
worth...a lot. Hey, lookee here my mood...I mean my faith ring has
turned green... Green, Hallelujah, my favorite denomination... So
load up the kids and come on down to Lloyd's... Remember at
"Lloyd's Holy World" you do the saving.

M. BUTTERFLY
by David Henry Hwang
A Paris prison - Present - Gallimard (65)

Gallimard is a man facing the fact that his life has been based on a lie. Sent to China as a diplomat, Gallimard began a 20 year love affair with the beautiful Song Liling, a popular opera singer who, in reality, was a spy...and a man. Unbelievably, Song's gender remained unknown to Gallimard, who allowed himself to fall in love with his fantasy of Asian women as personified in the character Madame Butterfly. Gallimard spends his days and nights in prison reviewing his past, and has concluded that he must kill himself in order to restore honor. Here, Gallimard prepares to commit a ritual hare kari.

GALLIMARD: I've played out the events of my life night after night, always searching for a new ending to my story, one where I leave this cell and return forever to my Butterfly's arms.

Tonight I realize my search is over. That I've looked all along in the wrong place. And now, to you, I will prove that my love was not in vain—by returning to the world of fantasy where I first met her.

(He picks up the kimono; dancers enter.)

GALLIMARD: There is a vision of the Orient that I have. Of slender women in chong sams and kimonos who die for the love of unworthy foreign devils. Who are born and raised to be the perfect women. Who take whatever punishment we give them, and bounce back, strengthened by love, unconditionally. It is a vision that has become my life.

(Dancers bring the wash basin to him and help him make up his face.)

GALLIMARD: In public, I have continued to deny that Song Liling is a man. This brings me headlines, and is a source of great embarrassment to my French colleagues, who can now be sent into a coughing fit by the mere mention of Chinese food. But alone, in my cell, I have long since faced the truth.

M. BUTTERFLY

And the truth demands a sacrifice. For mistakes made over the course of a lifetime. My mistakes were simple and absolute—the man I loved was a cad, a bounder. He deserved nothing but a kick in the behind, and instead I gave him...all my love.

Yes—love. Why not admit it all? That was my undoing, wasn't it? Love warped my judgment, blinded my eyes, rearranged the very lines on my face...until I could look in the mirror and see nothing but...a woman.

(Dancers help him put on the Butterfly wig.)

GALLIMARD: I have a vision. Of the Orient. That, deep within its almond eyes, there are still women. Women willing to sacrifice themselves for the love of a man. Even a man whose love is completely without worth.

(Dancers assist Gallimard in donning the kimono. They hand him a knife.)

GALLIMARD: Death with honor is better than life...life with dishonor. *(He sets himself center stage, in a seppuku position)* The love of a Butterfly can withstand many things—unfaithfulness, loss, even abandonment. But how can it face the one sin that implies all others? The devastating knowledge that, underneath it all, the object of her love was nothing more, nothing less than...a man. *(He sets the tip of the knife against his body.)* It is 1991. And I have found her at last. In a prison on the outskirts of Paris. My name is Rene Gallimard—also known as Madame Butterfly.

MAKING HISTORY
by Brian Friel
Ireland - 16th Century - Harry Hoveden (40's)

Harry is Hugh O'Neill's devoted secretary. When O'Neill, Earl of Tyrone, forms an alliance with Spain, war breaks out in Ireland. O'Neill and his men are forced into hiding. Harry has taken Mabel, O'Neill's pregnant wife, to a safe place. When Mabel dies in childbirth, Harry is faced with the painful task of telling O'Neill. As he tells his leader of his wife's death, he reveals that he, too has always loved Mabel.

HARRY: What else?... There's a rumour that Mountjoy himself may be in trouble because of some woman in England—Lady Penelope Rich?—is that the name? Anyhow if the scandal becomes public they say Mountjoy may be recalled. What else was there...? Sean na bPunta is still going calmly round the country with his brown leather bag, collecting your rents as if the place weren't in chaos!... Tadhg O Cianain is writing a book on the past ten years— [O'DONNELL: Another history! Jesus, if we had as many scones of bread as we have historians!]
HARRY: It will be a very exact piece of work that Tadhg will produce... And portions of another book are being circulated and it seems the English government is paying a lot of attention to it. Written by an Englishman called Spenser who used to have a place down near the Ballyhouras mountains—wherever they are—I'm getting like you, Hugh—they're in County Cork, aren't they?—anyhow this Spenser was burned out in the troubles after the battle of the Yellow Ford— *(He suddenly breaks down but continues speaking without stopping.)* Oh, my God, Hugh, I don't know how to say it to you—I don't know how to tell you—we had only just arrived at O Cathain's place—
[O'DONNELL: Harry—?]
HARRY: And the journey *had* been fine—she was in wonderful form—we sang songs most of the way—I taught her 'Tabhair Dom Do Lamh', Ruadhaire Dall's song, because the O Cathains are

54

relatives of his and she could show off before them and we laughed until we were sore at the way she pronounced the Irish words—and she taught me a Staffordshire ballad called 'Lord Brand, He was a Gentleman' and I tried to sing it in a Staffordshire accent—and she couldn't have been better looked after—they were all waiting for her—Ethna, the doctor O Coinne, two midwives, half-a-dozen servants. And everything seemed perfectly normal—everything *was* fine. She said if the baby was a boy she was going to call it Nicholas after her father and if it was a girl she was going to call it Joan after your mother—and when Ethna asked her were you thinking of going into exile she got very agitated and she said, 'Hugh?' She said, 'Hugh would never betray his people'—and just then, quite normally, quite naturally, she went into labour—and whatever happened—I still don't really know—whatever happened, something just wasn't right, Hugh. The baby lived for about an hour—it was a boy—but she never knew it had died—and shortly afterwards Ethna was sitting on a stool right beside her bed, closer than I am to you—and she was sleeping very peacefully—and then she gave a long sigh as if she were very tired and when Ethna put her hand on her cheek... It wasn't possible to get word to you—it all happened so quickly—herself and the baby within two hours—the doctor said something about poisoning of the blood— Oh, God, I'm so sorry for you—I'm so sorry for all of us. I loved her, too—you know that—from the very first day we met her—remember that day in May?—her twentieth birthday?—she was wearing a blue dress with a white lace collar and white lace cuffs... If you had seen her laid out she looked like a girl of fourteen, she was just so beautiful... God have mercy on her. God have mercy on all of us.

THE MOJO AND THE SAYSO
by Aishah Rahman
The Benjamins' home - Present - Blood (20's)

Blood is a young man struggling to come to terms with the accidental shooting death of his ten year-old brother. Vascillating between bouts of violence and despair, Blood here shares a memory of heartache with his father.

BLOOD: *(As he speaks he writes red graffiti on the new window panes)* I had a woman once. She worked at the express counter in the supermarket. I used to make seven, eight shopping trips a day just to walk through her line. Every time she saw me she smiled and I was sure she really loved me. Whenever she asked me if I wanted a single or double bag I knew she was really pledging her love. And all those times I replied, "Single bag, thank you" I was really asking her to let me drink her bathwater.

Although I never knew her name, we were very happy. All over the city I drew red hearts for her. No clean space went unmarked. I even added some of my blood to the red paint. When I pricked all my fingers and toes I started on my knuckles and ankles. It hurt like hell!

One time I stayed up all night making hearts for her. Next morning I ran to our supermarket and got on her line. Some man was with her making her laugh. She didn't even know that I was there. I just stood there looking at her. I screamed at her silently, "You love him and not me. You want his low voice, his strong chest and his big thighs. Why can't you want me?" I was very angry.

THE MOJO AND THE SAYSO
by Aishah Rahman
The Benjamins' home - Present - Acts (40-50)

Acts is a man working hard to hold his family together after the
tragic death of their youngest son. To him the task is rather like
restoring a classic car: something to be done with care and love.
When accused by his oldest son of never communicating his
feelings, Acts delivers the following monologue.

ACTS: Okay, you been after me all this time so I'm gonna talk.
Gonna tell you something. So listen real good.
*(As ACTS speaks, BLOOD keeps peeling, letting the peelings and
fruit pile up on the floor. Every once in a while he seems to nick
himself accidentally.)*
In this world, in order to survive, you gotta have a little gris-gris
to depend on. It could be anything. A prayer, a saying, a rabbit
foot, a horseshoe, a song. A way of looking at life, a way of doing
things, a way of understanding the world you find yourself in.
Something that will never fail to pull you through the hard times.
Now I see you got no formula for survival, no magic, no juju, so let
me give you a very important piece of mojo right now. Always
remember that the secret of a car is its engine. The engine is the
car's heart. Treat it right and you can trust it. The trick is you
gotta take your time and learn it. Study it inside out. Most folks
abuse the engine by racing it when it's cold. How would you like
to be waked up in the morning by someone shouting and screaming
at you while you're still yawning and under the covers? You
couldn't respond even if you wanted to. It takes time to fully warm
up. And you gotta give it good fuel. Then you gotta inspire it. Set
it on fire. Ignite the bad boy. Then he's gotta be stroked and
lubricated real good. Now don't forget there's plenty of fire and
heat inside so you gotta cool him off, too. Learn the engine, boy.
Understand the heart. It's the secret of life.

A POSTER OF THE COSMOS
by Lanford Wilson
New York City police station - 1987 - Tom (36)

When Tom is discovered in his lover's hospital room covered with blood, he is arrested for murder. Here, Tom begins his explanation to the police. When Johnny was diagnosed as HIV positive, Tom's own torment began as well. Even though Tom has remained AIDS-free, his desire to die with Johnny was strong enough to trigger his bloody act on Johnny's death bed.

TOM: All right, I'm sitting down and I'm staying down. Okay?
(He sits)
Now, are you happy?
(Glares at them in disgust)
Jesus, you guys slay me with that crap. "You don't look like the kinna guy'd do somethin' like dat." You're a joke. Cops. Jesus. I mean you're some total cliché. I don't have to be here lookin' at you guys, I could turn on the TV. "What's that white stuff on your shirt?" Jesus. I'm a baker, it's flour. You want a sample, take to your lab?
(Shaking his head in wonder)
"You don't look like the kinna guy..." What does dat kinna guy who'd do somethin' like dat look like to a cop, huh? And what kinna *thing?* You don't know nothin'; you know what you think you know. You seen every kinna dirty business there is every night, lookin' under the covers, spend your workin' day in the fuckin' armpits of the city and still ain't learned shit about people. You're totally fuckin' blind and deaf like fish I heard about, spend their life back in some fuckin' cave.
(He looks around, taps the tape recorder, looks at it)
Is this on? You got your video cameras goin'? 'Cause I told you I'd tell you but this is the only time I'm tellin' this. So, you know, get out your proper equipment, I'm not doin' this twice.
(He looks around, still disgusted)
"You don't look like the kinna guy'd do somethin' like dat."

58

A POSTER OF THE COSMOS

Johnny said I didn't look like no kinna guy at all. Just a big ugly guy. Said I was like Kurt Vonnegut or somebody. Somebody had the good sense not to look like nobody else. He said that, I read every word Vonnegut wrote. He's good. He's got a perverted point of view, I like that. There was a time I wouldn't of understood that, but we change, which is what I'm sayin' here.

(Beat)

"You don't look like the kinna guy'd do dat." What kinna guy is *that? What* kinna guy? Oh, well, you're talkin; *dat* kinna guy. The kinna guy'd *do* that. *Dat* kinna guy... Well, I *ain't* dat kinna guy. I'm a kinna guy like *you* kinna guys. That's why you make me want to puke sittin' here lookin' at you. "Hey, guys, dis guy is our kinna guy. I can't believe he's dat kinna guy." Well, I *ain't* that kinna guy.

RECKLESS
by Craig Lucas
Ohio and Alaska - Present - Fourth Doctor (30-50)

The chief suspect in a murder that she did not commit, Rachel lives her life on the run; constantly changeing towns and her name. She always manages to find the time to see a psychiatrist, however, and here one of their number attempts to induce in Rachel a primal scream.

FOURTH DOCTOR: This is very important, Cheryl. We've talked about the birth scream. It is a terrible shock to be torn away in a shower of blood with your mother screaming and your home torn open and the strange doctor with his rubber hands slapping you with all his might and the cold light piercing the dark, the warm beautiful wet dark, the silent murmuring safe dark of Mummy everywhere and Daddy, everything is one and everything is sex and we are all together for eternity and we are happy and nothing ever passes through your mind but good thoughts until suddenly this squeezing is going on around you and everyone is pushing and pulling and cold steel tongs pinch your skin and pull you by the top of your head and you don't want to go, no, you don't want to leave your home where you're always floating and your mother's heart is always beating for something unknown and cruel where people are cold and you're stinging now, everything is breaking, it makes you want to scream, Cheryl, makes you want to scream the scream of all ages, scream of the greatest tragedy of all time and your mummy is screaming and your daddy is screaming and now all the doctors are screaming and everything's blinding you and you're torn away and they're hitting you and they throw you up in air you open your eyes and your mother is covered in blood and you scream, Cheryl, scream, scream, *scream*, Cheryl, SCREAM, *SCREAM!!!* *(Pause.)* All right, we'll try it again.

THE SENATOR WORE PANTYHOSE
by Billy Van Zandt and Jane Milmore
New Jersey - Present - Gabby (40's)

"Honest" Gabby Sandalson is at the end of his political rope. His campaign for president has all but stripped his soul. To win the popular vote, Gabby has grudgingly allowed his campaign manager to darken his eyebrows, mousse his hair, introduce him to TV evangelists, and dress him in pantyhose. When an investigative reporter exposes Gabby's ploys, the good senator explodes with frustration in front of the TV camera and winds up with even more votes than he had before.

GABBY: *(To Tom.)* I don't want to be elected this way. I will not continue this charade.

[TOM: Don't do this!]

GABBY: *(Takes mike and speaks into camera.)* I tried. I really tried. I danced the Indian tribal dances, I ate chili, I moussed my hair, I wore makeup. On St. Patrick's Day I wore green and changed my name to Gabby O'Sandalson. But I can't go on like this. Look at me. Look at me! Look at my wife!

(SUSAN waves at the camera in a very First-Ladylike way.)

GABBY: What have I become? I don't want to be part of a system that elects people this way. It has to be honest. If it's not honest it's not worth it. The country has a lot of problems but they are never going to be solved unless we get our priorities straight. And our priorities shouldn't be what I look like, or how much I sweat, or what color my eyebrows are.

(Offstage BAND plays "Battle Hymn" under the following. The OTHERS hum. One by one, led by TOM, THEY begin marching in place, hands over their hearts. TOM waves flags.)

GABBY: George Washington was an ugly man with wooden teeth. John Adams was an ugly little shrimp with a bad attitude problem. Abraham Lincoln was a gawky doofus with massive facial hair. And a big hairy mole right here. *(Points to chin.)* But they were all great men! Today, none of them could even get elected.

THE SENATOR WORE PANTYHOSE

Somewhere along the way we lost our most important priority. The issues! I can't be president unless the people want me for who I am, and what I stand for. Don't cheat yourself out of a future looking for a gameshow host when what you need is a leader. Serving to uphold the Constitution, one nation, under God, indivisible, with liberty and justice for all!

THREE WAYS HOME
by Casey Kurtti
New York City - Present - Frankie (16)

Sharon fills a void in her life through a volunteer program, where she becomes involved with Dawn, an underprivileged, defensive black woman, and Dawn's sensitive but troubled teenaged son, Frankie. Here, Frankie tells the audience how he believes in the X-Men (comic book heroes) and identifies with them as mutants.

FRANKIE: Yo, what's up? My Mom's got all these people now, first James, then her psycho worker, now this new other one. Soon you're going to see the whole Secret Service pull up here and act as her damn body guard. I mean WORD, she's got all these people around her now I got to climb in the back seat? I used to be Numero Uno around here till James came on the scene. Dude shows up smack dab on my thirteenth birhtday. Ruins my whole life. 'Cause he got between me and my Moms. We used to be like this. But he messed up something that can't be put back together. Now I'm just supposed to hang around and do household chores? Yo, do I look like Mary Poppins to you? I got things to do, so let James watch the kids. I hate that guy. He doesn't do any thing anyway. Just leans on my ass. It's not like he's my damn father! It's because of him I can't stand it around here, so I'm changing things around... *(Pulls out an X-Men comic book)* ...See I'm modeling myself after the X-Men. You ever hear of them? I'll tell you a little bit about them. My older brothers and a couple of sisters started making their appearance around 1967 in a comic book about their lives. They're stationed on this here planet. Sometimes they travel to other worlds, secret locations, they're all mutants... Fucked up. Bent out of shape. But they're not just fucked up. They got some kick-ass powers. That's why after some serious research I hooked up with the X-Men. See, you got some sleeping creatures hiding in these here buildings. *(Leaps onto fire escapes.)* One time, three years ago, they tried to grab a hold of my sister Tawny. I saved her

THREE WAYS HOME

but they got a hold of my ass. They messed me up—tried to do me like a girl—so my Moms took me to this place where they ask you a lot of questions you don't want to explain. I went back twice. Then I cured myself. Started reading The X-Men and I learned how to get my guard up. *(Begins "acting out" Wolverine fantasy.)* See this here world fears them because they're different. I dig them cause they're not all good or bad. That's the way I am. Not all good or all bad. You dig? Well take Wolverine... Man... He's a hairy ass Mother Fucker with razor sharp claws. They're made of adamantium, that's the strongest metal known to mankind. Wolverine is all messed up in the face, but basically a very nice person. Sometimes I go over to Central Park and listen to my sounds. Think about them coming to life, making an appearance. To teach me about the powers. So I can prepare for my life, take care of James and some other things. They could show up one of these days. It's possible. Then I won't have to be alone. Learning all about life by myself. But I'm doing okay. Right now I'm teaching myself how to disappear. Check it out.

WHEN WE WERE WOMEN
by Sharman Macdonald
Scotland - During WWII - MacKenzie (20's-30's)

MacKenzie is a Chief Petty Officer in the Royal Navy stationed
at home during WWII. One evening he is caught outside during
a bombing raid. When the bombs begin to fall, MacKenzie hits
the dirt and begins to bargain with God for his life.

MACKENZIE: I'll get there if it damn well kills me.
Eh God. If you see what I've got waitin' for me you'd no send your
bombers in.

Our Father which are in Heaven,
I am a sinner.
Hallowed be thy name.
A terrible sinner.
Thy kingdom come.
I humbly ask.
Thy will be done.

Do not snuff me out. Me. God. Not me. I mean God. You're a
man. God. We're men together God. You and me. The pleasures
of the flesh eh. Soft flesh. Wrap you round. I bet you've had your
fling God. In your time. You've got to admit it. You were a one.
Eh? Eh? And now, eh? Stuck up there in your nice heaven what
have you got left. A pile of angels. There's no a lot you can do wi'
an angel. I mean when it comes right down to it. God. Looking
that's all you've got left. You're a bit of a voyeur.
(Bang.)
Mother Eve see to me. Mother Mary beloved of God hold me to thy
bosom.
(Bang.)
Perfumed skin. Powder. Red, red lips. Succour me.
(Bang.)
We're no gettin' very far here are we now. I mean look at me. A

65

WHEN WE WERE WOMEN

more foolish... Let me go. Come on. You let me go an' I'll sin
some more for your amusement God. Not bad sins when you come
right down to it. Wee sins in a minor key. When you consider
what could be done. There's a lot worse sinners than me... Aw,
come on, man... There's no bloody dignity in crawlin' along a wet
road on your belly.
(Bang.)

Give us this day our daily bread.

That's it. That's yer lot. I canny remember the rest of your prayer
God. God. Lord. Lord God. Let me off the rest of your prayer.
Give me one more day to breathe your crisp clean air.
*(Bang. He covers his head. Silence. The sound of crying. He lifts
his head.)*
You made me. You've got me. Take me or leave me as I am.
God. God.

WHEN WE WERE WOMEN
by Sharman Macdonald
Scotland - During WWII - Alec (50's)

Alec is an older man dancing with his daughter at her wedding.
As they spin around the dance floor, he offers advice on married
life and it is clear that his views reflect a more simple era when
life was a little less complicated.

ALEC: Dance wi' yer old man. Come to my arms wee hen.
(MAGGIE watches and sings on. ISLA and ALEC dance.) You'll
do well to let him be. I see your eyes. I know what you're
thinking. It's a wise woman that knows when to keep her mouth
shut. For a man to marry is a great thing. He's giving up
everything. A woman now that's a fair different story. A woman,
she gains everything. Position. A place in the eyes of the world.
On her finger for all to see she bears the mark of being wanted, the
mark of her belonging. A ring. It's what she's been brought up for.
The summit of her amibition. The goal of all her training. Look.
See him dancing there. Do they look well together? Aye, she can
dance. She can dance alright. Look how they move the both of
them. What if he strays. What if? You let him be. You smile an'
he'll come runnin' back. Mind me what I'm sayin' now. Mind.
These words are the gleanings of the years. I've learnt. I'm wise.
Oh yes I'm the wise one. Mind me. Mind what I'm sayin'. He's
a fine big man. An' you've caught him. That's a great thing. Now
you break him in gently. Be canny. Never nag. Give him that
much freedom he never knows he's been caught. Keep his meals hot
an' his bed well aired. Keep yersel' pure for him. An' mind you
wear some perfume on an evening. Mind that. There's nothing like
the smell of a woman's perfume. Mind all that an' he'll come home
to you and he'll bear with him armfuls of flowers an' a heart full of
gratitude that he'll lay at your feet. Gratitude'll hold a man longer
than any youthful idea of love. Gratitude's what makes a bond.
And guilt. I know. Do I not know. Love now. Love. That
merely makes the marriage. You smile my wee girl. Smile. Smile.
Let your beauty shine forth on this glorious day. For you've made
your old Father a happy, happy man.

ZERO POSITIVE
by Harry Kondoleon
Upper West Side apartment - 1987 - Patrick (30's)

Patrick is invited for lunch at his friend, Himmer's apartment. During the course of their conversation, Patrick reveals his frustration with his career and the powerful and greedy people who control it.

PATRICK: They are the devils. The evil devils. I swear on your mother's grave, devils walk the earth and they pray to their greedy god called Personal Gain and everything is sacrificed to its big fat mouth. Now, I'm an actor so I don't know your career but you can make an analogy to your experience at *Life*, everything is cutthroat, I know that, I'm not getting special bad treatment. But there are certain arenas where one is led to suspect beauty of spirit will rule the day and if not why then do the devils that tread there pick such a puny arena to pitch their tents? *What a bright nice fire!* I'll say when I watch them burn. And I will. I'll come back from the dead if I have to chew on the devils' throats... I cannot get a job, I cannot get a job.

ACAPULCO
by Steven Berkoff
Acapulco Plaza Hotel - Present - Will (30's)

Will is an actor working on location in Acapulco. Here, Will
joins Steve, a fellow actor, at the hotel bar and tries to start up
a conversation.

WILL: I just came in the bar... I was walking past... I thought.
'Shall I go in or not?'... And you're here! I didn't work today. I
didn't know what to do...I didn't feel like going to the beach at La
Questa. I just didn't feel like it... I felt out of it... Like I didn't
deserve it... I would have loved it...I mean, I love it down there,
but I just hung around this awful beach. Just walked up and down
and then I went downtown for a coffee. I felt desperate. Like out
of it. You went to La Questa! Was it beautiful there? Did you see
the sunset? You just sit and can meditate for hours. Stare at those
great breakers rolling in. No tourists. No Americans down there.
Just peace. You went down there, eh? I nearly went. I got up...
Looked at the day, but felt I didn't deserve it. I felt out of it, so I
walked around and had a coffee... And was walking back when I
thought, 'Why not try the bar?'... And you're here! Great! That
chick you were speaking to. She's a cock-teaser. I saw her in the
pool yesterday, and she smiled and came on strong like she was into
me. You know, she lightly touched my thigh as she spoke...in the
pool... I just dived in and as I surfaced there she was... You know,
I haven't been with a woman in three weeks. Like...this is
Acapulco. You know what I'm saying. Not even been out with
one... I had a hard-on and I wanted to put it somewhere. And then
I saw her talking to the other guys like I was just a piece of
furniture... I came out of my hotel this morning...you know...to get
a coffee...and that stunt guy was walking in the coffee shop with
four chicks! Four! I couldn't believe it...four of them. You know
your mind plays tricks. Fantasies of having the four...one at a
time... So I followed him to the coffee shop and listened at a
discreet distance... And what a piece of shit I heard... And I

69

immediately went off them. Somehow, you know, when you hear the stark reality of their minds. I felt repulsed. I couldn't go near them, so I felt down. I was walking past and I thought, 'Why not come in here?'... And, like magic... You know, you're the only person that I can relate to...in the whole fuckin' film... The others! The guy playing the sergeant... Fuck him...and the fuckin' stand-in! I walked past her trailer one morning and she looked nice. You know...kind of pretty, so I said, 'Hey! You're looking real pretty today' and do you know what she said? 'Oh, gimme a break.' I was just being friendly... She thinks because I'm playing a POW that I'm scum... 'Cause I was cast in Mexico and not in Hollywood. And 'cause I'm paid in pesos I'm scum... 'Cause we look like scum... Locked up in the wooden cage like some kind of animals... You know, this is such a goyish picture... There's not a Jew in the whole company except me...and, of course, you. But we're not like Jews...not like those Jews who worry all the time and are accountants... We're tough... I'm a tough Brooklyn Jew and they know it... You know... They can't mess around with me. You are tough, too! You came off the streets, right? Stallone's tough, but underneath you know Stallone's a very vulnerable guy. He's an Italian. The Jews and the Italians get on. What did you do today?

Steve, in turn, is a moody Brit who has just returned from an
unsuccessful sexual encounter with a young woman. When
Wills askes him about his day, he launches into a philosophical
and somewhat psychedelic accounting of his day's activities.

STEVE: I've not been to the John in the whole of Mexico... I wait
and hold it until I get back to the hotel... It stinks here... Everything stinks... So I went out to La Questa and saw the sunset...
The clouds moved slowly...bloody...at the edges...like cotton-wool
seeping slowly...like a knife had stabbed a big belly of a cloud...and
it was slowly going pink and then red... I went walking back in the
dark... There were huge craters in the road from the hurricane, so
I walked a bit. And the sky was like shrieking and the clouds were
bolting home looking ragged and torn...and there was a lagoon on
one side and sea on the other...and the sea was all rough but the
lagoon was like a sheet of glass. I walked and there was junk
everywhere... Mounds of old rotting coconuts and fruit that had
been left to the pigs... And the lizards were flicking in and out as
I passed near them... I heard them scrambling away as they felt my
footsteps... And I came to the end and there was a forest... You
know, like a jungle on one side with tall palms and some dirty old
huts and a few tables where you could eat and the kids were
swimming around in the sunset...
[WILL: Oh, the sunsets are beautiful!]
STEVE: You know...on the road there, there is a man with one leg
selling water mixed with some fruit juice...just standing there all day
and I didn't see him sell anything...all those large bottles.
[WILL: There's every juice in the world there...anything...and you
can drink the water.]
STEVE: At the end there's a café called Steve's Place...and you can
sit there and drink and watch the sunset. Flies buzzing around the
kitchen. All open... Dogs and cats sniffing around... Somebody's

71

ACAPULCO

always eating something indescribable.   But the fish was great!
Under the palm umbrella I had the red snapper.   It was laid out on
the plate like an offering...surrounded by sliced tomatoes and onions
and under a napkin were hot tortillas made out of flour...   No, they
were made from corn.   And it was on a tray.   And, as I looked at
the sea tearing itself into little pieces against the sand, I prised a
piece of fish off with my fork, which pulled away easily, beautifully
cooked, and wrapped it in the hot tortilla, perched a tomato on it,
onions, and folded it, and then added some salsa.   That hot sauce
that goes straight for the exit and misses out the middle man.   It
burns a road right through you.   So I sat and shooed the flies and
excavated the fish until I left the bones and the head and was careful
not to get too close to that thing...   But two little kids came and
asked for the head like it was a luxury for them.   They broke it off
the spine of the fish and chewed into it, eyes and all.   Boy! They
were so happy, they were laughing and chewing the head, since it
tasted good to them.   They were looking at me and laughing as if I
had been stupid and thrown away a great treat.   It looked really
disgusting with its eyes open.   Then a dog chewed the bones that
they left and then...I saw columns of ants descend on the crumbs...
The sun was, by this time, slowly sinking into the sea...like the
weight of it was too much.   It sank like a swollen bloated
belly...bulging even more as it sank.   Then scorched the sea up and
plunged down deep...   So I paid and left and walked a while.
Meanwhile, the little cafés were lit up with their kitchens all open
and frying and cooking and chopping tops off coconuts and this guy
had this really sharp machete and sliced the top off the coconut like
he was taking off a skull and I drank it.   It tasted sweet and strange.
Then I got a cab and came back.   The sunset was gorgeous.
Yeah...like a multi-coloured tropical flower...or like you took a huge
sword and stabbed the sea and it spewed blood everywhere with
drips hanging off the clouds.

ARCHANGELS DON'T PLAY PINBALL
by Dario Fo
translated by Ron Jenkins
Here and Now - Tiny (30's)

Hapless Tiny is accostomed to playing the fool for his friends
and is often the butt of the cruel jokes that they perpetrate. A
disabled vet, Tiny here shows a rare flash of anger when he
travels to Washington to collect his overdue pension. Rather
than submit to the snail-paced bureaucracy of the Veteran's
Administration, Tiny takes the entire building hostage.

TINY: Enough! Silence!... I said that's enough! Silence!
Enough! Shut up! *(Locks the door with a key.)* Now that I finally
have the honor of your full attention...listen to me!!!! I've come
here on very important business: my pension. I brought everything
with me... *(Opens the suitcase. Takes out a large packet of
documents, and deposits a pile under each one of the clerks' heads.)*
Birth certificates...residence papers...discharge papers...unlimited
liability   insurance...declaration   of   permanent   disability...
authorization forms...duplicates of the authorization forms...
triplicates of the authorization forms...carbon copy orginals of the
authorization forms. I don't understand any of them, but I did my
duty, now you do yours: verify them, sign them, stamp them. Put
on the seals, the counter-seals, the stamps, and the counter-stamps...
All I want to do is to leave here with the proper papers to get my
pension. *(He grabs the rubber stamps hanging from elastic cords
around the necks of each of the clerks, and attaches them to their
foreheads. Then he moves to the side of the windows and grabs a
lever which is attached to the counter on which he has placed all his
papers to be stamped.)* I've got no time to lose... And to make my
intentions clear, I brought a little something with me from Africa,
that I swear I'll set off if any of your tries to get smart with me.
Take a look: a model 38 hand grenade. *(He takes a bomb out of his
suitcase and puts it on the doorman's table. He begins shouting
commands.)* Round rubber stamps. *(Two clerks respond by lower-*

ARCHANGELS DON'T PLAY PINBALL

ing their heads to stamp his papers.) Square stamps. *(Two other clerks obey.)* All stamps. Stamp. Stamp. Stamp. Stamp, stamp, stamp. All stamps. *(The clerks do not obey.)* All stamps. *(They still don't obey.)* Damn. It's stuck. *(He pulls on the lever, trying to force it down. When he succeeds the counter begins to shake rhythmically, up and down under the noses of the clerks, whose foreheads, equipped with rubber stamps, bob up and down in alternating rhythms as they stamp the bouncing documents. It all gives the impression of an extraordinary futuristic machine.)* Stamp, stamp, stamp, stamp. *(As the rhythm builds, the action transforms itself into a steam engine that chugs along with a final "toot-toot" as it grinds to a stop.)* Toot-toot...ding, ding. We made it. And now all we need is my registration card which we'll find in my personal file. *(One wall is covered with filing drawers. TINY pulls out the one that interests him.)* The A's are here. S's over there. This must be the T's. Here it is. *(Puts the drawer under the face of the first clerk.)* Go on, find the file for Mr. Weather. First name Sunny, Cloudy, Stormy and first one who laughs get a bomb up his nose. *(The clerk picks out the file with his teeth. TINY narrates the search as if he were a game show host.)* It's the wheel of fortune. Round and round the clerk's mouth goes, but where it stops, nobody knows. Can he do it. Yes, that's it. He's hit the jackpot. It's me. Weather, Sunny, date of birth, distinguishing features...race: Labrador Retriever... No?!!.. Yes, that's what it says...race: Labrador Retriever...profession: hunter of birds: stunted tail: floppy ears, small teeth, apparently a mongrel... Ha Ha. *(Laughs hysterically.)* Apparently a mongrel?! *(The clerks laugh. TINY grabs the bomb and removes the safety pin. The clerks stop laughing.)* Whose idea was it to play this stinking trick on me? Come on, who was it? I warned you not to make fun of me. Not to play around. I don't even let my friends make a fool of me anymore, and they used to pay me for it... A labrador retriever, eh? *(Lifts up his arm to throw the bomb.)* This will teach you. Go on, laugh. Laugh for the last time. Laugh. Ha, ha ha. *(The clerks would like to shout for help, but are struck mute with terror. TINY spins around, playing with the bomb as if it were on a wheel of fortune.)* Place your bets, folks. Round and round the little bomb goes and where it lands, nobody knows...ha...ha...ha.

ARCHANGELS DON'T PLAY PINBALL
by Dario Fo
translated by Ron Jenkins
Here and Now - Tiny (30's)

Tiny has been set up in a fake wedding by his friends, who only desire to play yet another joke on their personal jester. Tiny believes that his veiled bride is, in fact, Angela, a woman whom he loves. Unveiled, the "bride" is revealed as an ugly specimen. Enraged, Tiny finally turns on his friends and then on Heaven itself.

TINY: *(Panting, trying to compose himself.)* Excuse me, but I've got nothing against you. If you're not beautiful, it's certainly not your fault. It's just that these sons of... *(Short pause.)* You're a professional, so I'm sure you understand. *(Walks downstage.)* But most of all, I'm fed up with whomever's in charge of manufacturing dreams. *(Almost speaking to the balcony.)* I want to know who's got that job. Which one of you archangels is it. Gabriel?... Michael?... Rapheal?... Who is it... *(He speaks as if he sees each one of them in the theater.)* Speak up, you archangels. If it's true what they told me when I was a child, that the Lord put you in charge of dream-making, why did you have to come and pick on me?... Giving me dreams with double meanings...why?... Now I'm going to start screaming such filthy curses that you'll have to plug up your ears with corks... Because if we can't even believe in our dreams any more... *(Shouting.)* ...then there's nothing left...it's the pits...it's the god awful shit in the hole pits... *(With a tense voice.)* What the hell do you think I am. A goddamn pinball machine that you can put your money in and bang around to make yourselves feel important?

THE AUTHOR'S VOICE
by Richard Greenberg
Todd's apartment - Present - Todd (20-30)

Unknown to everyone, Todd's best-selling novel was really
written by Gene, a pathetic gnome whom Todd has rescued from
the street. Todd and Gene quarrel violently when Gene sneaks
out of the apartment to go shopping. Here, Todd begs for
Gene's forgiveness and reveals his feelings of isolation.

TODD: Christ, I'm sorry! *(A beat.)* I didn't mean to hurt you.
Please come out. *(A beat.)* Please come out. *(A beat.)* I'm not a
cruel person. I'm not... I don't... *(A beat. The keening subsides)*
Gene? *(It starts again)* Gene, I'm sorry, I'm sorry, I'm sorry, I'm
sorry, I'm... *(He is now almost climbing the door, almost caressing
it, pacifying)* Listen... Listen... Listen... Gene? Gene?...
Gene?... *(The keening subsides again)* Gene, are you all right,
now? *(A beat, still quiet.)* Are you better? *(Still quiet)* Are you
better? *(Still quiet)* You sound better Gene, what can we do? Can
we be friends? Can we...? *(A beat)* Gene, listen, I'm going to do
like we used to, okay? Remember? I'm going to tell you something
that happened to me and you can tell me what it means, remember?
Okay? *(A beat)* Is that okay? *(A beat)* Is that okay? *(A beat)*
Okay. *(He sits with his back against the door.)* This happened the
other day at the Health Club. You know, where I go? *(A beat)*
Right. Well, I was going to take a swim. I'd never used the pool
there before, but I wanted to swim. So I was getting suited up when
a man at the row of lockers across from me started talking to his
friend. This man, he was balding, but he seemed pretty fit, and he
was pleased with himself, you could tell, like he didn't even mind
being bald, and I thought, well, if I feel like that at his age, I won't
be doing half bad. And his friend looked pretty good, too, and it
sort of cheered me up. Anyway, they went to the pool. I finished
getting ready, and then I went to the pool. It was just the three of
us and an attendant. The attendant yelled at me, "No trunks!" I
didn't understand. Then I looked at the two men swimming in the

pool. They were naked. It was policy. When they were naked like that, they didn't look so good. They looked fat. They looked like fish—large...extinct...fish... I bent to take off my trunks. As I did, the bald man came up for air. For a second, he was completely still, frozen solid in the water. He looked at me and kept looking. I dove in, a perfect dive with a flip and a spin. When I came up for air, the bald man wasn't in the pool any more. He was standing by the poolside, crying hysterically. His friend was next to him, trying to calm him down, but the bald-headed man wouldn't stop crying. "Why are you crying?" his friend kept asking. "It was the dive." he said. "It was the dive." *(A beat)* Gene...? *(A beat)* Gene, why did that make him cry? *(A beat)* Why?... Why did that make him cry? *(A beat)* Gene...? Gene...? Why?

[GENE: *(From the bedroom; braying)* BECAUSE IT WAS SAD! *(A beat)*]

TODD: Oh. *(A beat)* I need you to tell me these sorts of things, Gene. I can't figure them out on my own. *(A beat)* My life isn't good. You think it is, but it's not. Once it was, but it's not any more. *(A beat)* I used to be made happy by...stupid things. Parties! People around me. I was vain. I was a peacock. I looked in the mirror. I looked so hard I didn't recognize myself. I didn't recognize anything. I forgot why I did things. I got scared, Gene! I got scared outside, I got scared in my room. I didn't know where I was half the time. I wanted to drown, I wanted to be covered over... Then I found you. *(A beat)* Make me famous, Gene. I want to be famous. People will photograph me and write about me. I'll study how they see me and live inside it... Fame will be a kind of home. But I need you to get it for me. Only they can't know it's you, they can't know it's *you*; if they ever see you, it will die like *that*. *(Snaps his fingers. A beat)* It panics me when you leave and it panics me when you're here. You're the whole problem of my life, but without you I don't have any life. *(A beat)* I'll give you what you want. I won't deny you any more. Anything I can, I'll give you.

EMERALD CITY
by David Williamson
Sydney, Australia - Present - Colin (30's)

When Colin is offered the opportunity to produce a soap opera, he jumps at it. When his wife suggests that a soap opera isn't exactly a worthy showplace for his talents, he explains his motivation.

COLIN: *(suddenly, passionately)* What's happening is that I'm getting older and I'm starting to have the nightmare that every writer gets: ending my life as a deadbeat, flogging scripts to producers who don't want 'em. And it's not paranoia. It happens. Henry Lawson was sent to jail in the street of Sydney and did anyone care? Not one. He'd be really amused today if he could see his head on our ten dollar note. Cultural hero—kids study him in schools—ended his life as a joke and nobody cared! It's not going to happen to me. I'm sick of sending scripts off and waiting patiently for the call that never comes and ringing back and ringing back and finally getting someone on the other end of the phone who says, "Sorry," they haven't had time to read it yet. Being a writer is one of the most humiliating professions on earth and I'm sick to death of it. I want to be a producer, and I want to have money, and I want to have power. I want to sit in my office with people phoning *me*. I want to sit back and tell my secretary that I'm in conference and can't be disturbed and that I'll ring back, then make sure I never do. I want scripts to come to *me*, and *I'll* make the judgements about whether they're good bad or indifferent. *I'll* be the one with the blue pencil who rips other people's scripts apart, complains about the banality and predictability, groans at the clichéd dialogue, mutters, "There must be some good writers *somewhere*." Why *shouldn't* I have money and power? Why *shouldn't* I have a great big house on the waterfront like all the rest of the coked-out mumblers out there masquerading as producers? I want *you* to stop telling people what *I* want out of *my* life, because you are *wrong*! I don't want to make art films or films with a message, I want to produce a product that entertains and I want it to make me awesomely powerful and fabulously rich!

79

FRANKIE AND JOHNNY IN THE CLAIR DE LUNE
by Terrence McNally
New York City - Present - Johnny (30-40)

On their first date, Frankie and Johnny return to Frankie's apartment for a round of passionate lovemaking. Johnny is clearly smitten with Frankie, who can't seem to overcome her fear of becoming emotionally connected. When he finally declares his love for her, she orders him to leave. Instead of leaving, Johnny phones the radio station that they've been listening to and makes the following request.

JOHNNY: *(Into phone.)* May I speak to your disc jockey?... Well excuse me! *(He covers phone, to Frankie.)* They don't have a disc jockey. They have someone called Midnight With Marlon. *(Into phone.)* Hello, Marlon? My name is Johnny. My friend and I were making love and in the afterglow, which I sometimes think is the most beautiful part of making love, she noticed that you were playing some really beautiful music, piano. She was right. I don't know much about quality music, which I could gather that was, so I would like to know the name of that particular piece and the artist performing it so I can buy the record and present it to my lady love, whose name is Frankie and is that a beautiful coincidence or is it not? *(Short pause.)* Bach. Johann Sebastian, right? I heard of him. The Goldberg Variations. Glenn Gould. Columbia Records. *(To Frankie.)* You gonna remember this? *(Frankie smacks him hard across the cheek. Johnny takes the phone from his ear and holds it against his chest. He just looks at her. She smacks him again. This time he catches her hand while it is still against his cheek, holds it a beat, then brings it to his lips and kisses it. Then, into phone, he continues but what he says is really for Frankie, his eyes never leaving her.)* Do you take requests, Marlon? Then make an exception! There's a man and a woman. Not young, not old. No great beauties, either one. They meet where they work: a restaurant and it's not the Ritz. She's a waitress. He's a cook. They meet but they don't connect. "I got two medium burgers working" and "Pick up, side of fries" is pretty much the extent of it. But she's noticed him, he can feel it. And he's noticed her. Right off. They both knew tonight was going to happen. So why did it take him six weeks for him to ask her if she wanted to see a movie that neither one of them could tell you the name of right now? Why did they eat ice cream sundaes before she asked him if he wanted to come up since they were in the neighborhood? And then they were making love and for maybe an hour they forgot the ten million things that made them think "I don't love this person. I don't even like them" and instead all they knew was that they were together and it was perfect and they were perfect and that's all there was to know about it and as they lay there, they both began the million reasons not to love one another like a familiar rosary. Only this time he stopped himself. Maybe it was the music you were playing. They both heard it. Only now they're both beginning to forget they did. So would you play something for Frankie and Johnny on the eve of something that ought to last, not self-destruct. I guess I want you to play the most beautiful music ever written and dedicate it to us. *(He hangs up.)*

INDIGO
by Heidi Thomas
Africa and West Indies - 1790's - Samuel (50's)

Samuel Randall is a British merchant who has made his fortune in the slave trade. Samuel's morality is constantly attacked by his son, William. Here, he takes a moment to reflect upon the events that led to his decision to become a slaver.

SAMUEL: When our William was a babby I was working with my hands. Samuel Randall, Master Ropemaker. I had calluses like you'd never believe. Stubborn ochre finger—skin, crusted white, as horny as a goat's hoof. But I was proud. I bore them hands with a high heart. The stigmata of the skilled peasantry. "It's an honest living," I would say. "An honest living." His mother bathed him once in a bowl upon the hearthstone. The water washed red in the firelight. Red and gold. He was that bonny, plump and tender like a pink peeled chestnut...

(He stops short.)

I said, "Give him to me, Mary Ann," and she did as she were bid. "There's my babba, there's my son." But he kicked with his feet and started crying. "What's the matter, lad?" I said. "Dost not like thy dadda, then?" Then I saw what it was. It was my hands. Gravelly scab-gritted hands blighting unbroken babyskin. "There," I said. "There is the price of an honest living." And I swore to myself that the same fate would not come to William. A man could be held underwater by hands like those. A man could drown of a life like that. So I started swimming. I began to fight. And I didn't care whose coat-tails I clutched onto or whose gasping head I trod on as I scrambled for the air. I had struggled enough. To breathe was beautiful.

INDIGO
by Heidi Thomas
Africa and West Indies - 1790's - Ide (20's)

Ide is an African prince whose father has chosen to deal with the European slave traders. When Ide hears tales of Christianity, he is struck by the concept of a god who sends his only son out into the world. Ide decides to allow himself to be sold as a slave so that he can lead his people to freedom. Here, he performs one last tribal ceremony.

IDE: I leave him behind. The man who was there at my bursting into being. At my earliest cry. At my first faint milk-eyed searching for the sun. There will always be the light trail laid between us; childhood touches like a chain of shadows, adult words like a crooked fence of sticks. Little broken images go hand in retreating hand. I turn, exultant, to the power that created me. The one god who begat me. One god, omnipotent. My father.
(He takes the incense and begins to swirl it over the coals.)
You cupped the elements in your hands; leaves and water; blood and flowers; salt and hair. Flesh-speckled motes of being, fine as grain. You ran them like sand through your fingers. I fell to ground and was formed like a weather-sculpted stone; with salt-white coral of my bones to support me and rich skin to ripple like a midnight sea. The sky is a sheet of semen, ruched by your sacred hands and held up high. I curve with the brown earth, sweep with the river's path, swell like a gourd in the rain! Tongue my body with your thread of flame. Raise my head to your radiant heat. Give me the strength to be your son and guide my exiled people where they did not wish to go...

LAUGHING WILD
by Christopher Durang
Here and Now - Man (30's)

A man addresses the audience from a podium. He begins by
telling of his experience in a personality workshop and of his
daily battle with negativity. He then breaks from his prepared
speech and recounts an unpleasant encounter he recently
experienced in a grocery store.

MAN: *(Off the cards again.)* And it is hard for me to be positive
because I'm very sensitive to the vibrations of people around me, or
maybe I'm just paranoid. But in any case, I used to find it difficult
to go out of the house sometimes because of coming into contact
with other people.

You've probably experienced something similar—you know, the
tough on the subway who keeps staring at you and you're the only
two people in the car and he keeps staring and after a while you
think, does he want to kill me? Or just intimidate me? Which is
annoying enough.

Or the people in movie theaters who talk endlessly during the
opening credits so you can just *tell* they're going to talk through the
entire movie and that it will be utterly useless to ask them not to
talk.

And even if you do ask them not to talk and they ungraciously
acquiesce, they're going to send out vibrations that they hate you all
during the entire film, and then it will be impossible to concentrate.

You can move, but the person next to you in the new location
will probably, you know, rattle candy wrappers endlessly all through
the movie. Basically I don't go to the movies anymore. What's the
point?

But even if you can skip going to the movies, you pretty much
have to go to the supermarket.

(Steps closer to the audience.) I was in the supermarket the
other day about to buy some tuna fish when I sensed this very
disturbed presence right behind me. There was something about her

84

focus that made it very clear to me that she was a disturbed person. So I thought—well, you should never look at a crazy person directly, so I thought, I'll just keep looking at these tuna fish cans, pretending to be engrossed in whether they're in oil or in water, and the person will then go away. But instead *wham!* she brings her fist down on my head and screams: "Would you move asshole!" *(Pause.)*

Now why did she do that? She hadn't even said, "Would you please move" at some initial point, so I would've known what her problem was. Admittedly I don't always tell people what I want either—like the people in the movie theaters who keep talking, you know, I just give up and resent them—but on the other hand, I don't take my fist and go wham! on their heads!

I mean, analyzing it, looking at it in a positive light, this woman probably had some really horrible life story that, you know, kind of explained how she got to this point in time, hitting me in the supermarket. And perhaps if her life—*since birth*—had been explained to me, I could probably have made some sense out of her action and how she got there. But even with that knowledge—which I didn't have—it was *my* head she was hitting, and it's just so unfair.

It makes me want to never leave my apartment *ever ever again. (Suddenly he closes his eyes and moves his arms in a circular motion around himself, round and round, soothingly.)*

MIXED FEELINGS
by Donald Churchill
England - Present - Harold (40's)

Arthur lives downstairs from Norma, his ex-wife, who is currently living with Harold, his best friend. When Norma tells Arthur that she no longer loves Harold, she pleads with him to break the bad news to his friend so she will be spared such a noisome chore. When the blow is dealt, Harold feels betrayed by both Arthur and Norma.

HAROLD: Where is the double-crossing rat?

[SONIA: Which rat are you referring to?]

HAROLD: Arthur! The man whose life I saved in 1959 in St. Anton.

[SONIA: I don't know about that.]

HAROLD: That's how we first met. I was skiing in Austria and I stopped Arthur going over a two-hundred foot crevasse by throwing myself in his path. He got a bruise, I got a broken ankle, and what do I get thirty years later?

[SONIA: Do I get a *little* clue, Harold?]

HAROLD: I got my arse kicked! *(HE goes down to the kitchen and starts looking for a glass.)* You want a clue! No one ever gave me the slightest hint. *(HE pours himself a drink.)* Don't you think I should have been put in the picture a little earlier? Be fair Sonia. I travel five thousand miles through mosquito infested jungle, down rivers full of crocodiles, piranhas and poisonous water snakes. I get mugged in Lima, mugged in Bogota, get strip searched in New York, strip searched in London, cheated by the cab driver who brought me from Heathrow. I finally arrive home and my bags are packed! No surprise to anyone but me! Everyone has known for weeks that Norma was going to chuck me out, but me. You'd expect something a bit better than that from... *(The drink and the emotion makes HIS voice tremble.)* ...your oldest friend. In wet weather my ankle still twinges. I let him break my ankle and he does this to me. *(Bursts into tears. SONIA goes to comfort him but stops herself.)* He could have tipped me the wink a bit earlier. Is that unreasonable, Sonia?

NIEDECKER
by Kristine Thatcher
Rural Wisconsin - 1963 - Al (50's)

Al is an earthy man who has spent his life as a physical laborer. Al has come to Rock River, Wisconsin to do some fishing. There he meets Lorine, a poetess who he falls in love with and marries. Here, Al tells Lorine of the fine art of catching pike.

AL: [Any kind. Don't matter. But] if you're looking for real adventure, there's nothing like going to get yourself a northern, nothing like it.

[LORINE: I've heard they're real fighters.]

AL: They're maniacs! Best bait in the world is frog—you slip the hook in his back, see, just under the spine, so he can swim free once he's in the water. When you've got him secure—and if you don't have much experience, it's a messy job, you've got to learn to do it clean—you cast that devil out as far as you can. Set your brake. Then, if you put the butt end of the rod in a piece of pipe on the shore and slip a tin can over the top of it, you're free to go about building a fire, taking a snooze, whatever you want; until you hear that can pop off the top of that pole. When you hear it go clattering, it's time to grab up the rod as fast as you can. The first order of business is setting the hook, and that's just a question of feel, learning when the fish is going for the heart of the frog. With a well-timed snap of the wrist, you can guarantee that fish a place on your supper table. But a northern pike is a fighter, a mean son of a bitch, who runs deep. You've got to play him just right or he'll snap your line. It's a matter of pulling back, reeling in, and easing off when you have to. At the very last, he'll come head first out of the water fighting mad, not like a trout or salmon, who ride their tails. It's the mouth that scares you.

[LORINE: Why?]

AL: Because a pike has a long snout and a top and bottom row of jagged teeth. Just when you think you can net him, he'll run at you again, so it looks like a damned alligator lunging up the line. Strikes terror into the heart.

87

PENGUIN BLUES
by Ethan Phillips
Alcohol rehab center - Present - Gordon (35)

When Gordon is asked to welcome Sister Angelita to the rehab
center, he greets her nervously, his fear of nuns—even one who
is a fellow alcoholic—giving way to foolish banter about balding.

GORDON: I'm losing all my hair. Rip-off. I was going to this
woman in L.A....uhh...who's supposed to make it grow again.
Jesus Christ. Dumb treatment. She's got this dumb treatment thing
she does, it costs like sixty bucks a shot, she squeezes this lemon
citrus solution on the scalp, and then rubs it in really hard, and it
stings, she's this French woman, and it really stings like it's on fire,
and then she puts "special mud" on it, which kind of cools it off a
little, and you sit there with this mud on your head for twenty
minutes and there's all these other women in the room, you know,
her other clients, getting their eyelashes dyed or something, and
talking about shoes and stuff and you feel like an idiot sitting there.
And then finally she washes it off, and then she takes this electronic
comb, it has this, umm...have you ever seen those electronic fly
catchers, those electric grill-like boxes with a zappy blue light that
kills flies? When they fly into it?
(Pause)
[ANGELITA: No.]
GORDON: This comb, it's the same kind of thing, this static blue
light...uhh, electricity that kind of pops when she scrapes it across
your scalp, and she just rakes this comb over your head and it really
hurts, you feel like punching her, and then she takes a regular comb
and combs around your hair and she always goes, "Ooh...I see all
these little bébé hairs coming up," but it's all bullshit 'cause I'm still
losing my hair and I'm out three thousand bucks from seeing this
woman, the only thing is I don't have any flies on my scalp, bit fat
deal.

PENGUIN BLUES
by Ethan Phillips
Alcohol rehab center - Present - Gordon (35)

Here, Gordon is finally able to reveal the source of his fear of nuns to patient Angelita.

GORDON: She... I was staying after school one day...in eighth grade... I was being punished for something... I can't remember what. And she told me to go down to the principal's office to get something or deliver something or something...and I was running down the hallway, feeling pretty good, believe it or not, and I tripped—my sneaker had a hole in it—and I tripped and hurt my knee when I fell—and I got real mad 'cause I was in a football game the next day and now my knee hurt, so I tore off the sneaker and started to rip it apart, I was really mad, and I said, "Shit. Fuck." And there, standing over me were these two nuns, and they heard me say, "shit, fuck" and they just looked at me and then they walked away, but I knew by the way they looked at me they were gonna tell Sister John and the next day was Saturday and football went okay and on Sunday I went to the children's mass and I'd been scared all weekend, but when I saw the look on Sister John's face at that mass, I was terrified. On Monday I was an angel all morning. I wasn't taking any chances. And then standing in line to go to lunch, in front of me was my best friend, Howie Jackson, and we used to do this thing—it was a silly little thing—I'd blow on the back of his neck and he'd kind of slap it, like that.
(Gordon slaps his neck, lightly)
I don't know where we got it from, but we used to do it all the time and it always made us smile, and I smiled and she saw me and that was all she needed...and this pig from hell came over and slapped me very hard, but she kept slapping me...in front of everyone...she just kept slapping me...and slapping me...and slapping me...she wouldn't stop...and I was just a little boy.

ROOSTERS
by Milcha Sanchez-Scott
Southwest - Present - Gallo (40's)

Gallo has spent the last several years in jail for manslaughter. Upon his release, he returns to his Chicano family in the southwest. His first visit, however, is to Zapata, the rooster that he bred and trained to fight in the ring. His love for the bird is nearly romantic, as can be seen in their first encounter.

GALLO: Lord Eagle, Lord Hawk, sainted ones, spirits and winds, Santa María Aurora of the Dawn... I want no resentment, I want no rancor... I had an old red Cuban hen. She was squirrel-tailed and sort of slab-sided and you wouldn't have given her a second look. But she was a queen. She could be thrown with any cock and you would get a hard-kicking stag every time.

I had a vision, of a hard-kicking flyer, the ultimate bird. The Filipinos were the ones with the pedigree Bolinas, the high flyers, but they had no real kick. To see those birds fighting in the air like dark avenging angels...well like my father use to say, "Son nobles...finos..." I figured to mate that old red Cuban. This particular Filipino had the best. A dark burgundy flyer named MacArthur. He wouldn't sell. I began borrowing MacArthur at night, bringing him back before dawn, no one was the wiser, but one morning the Filipino's son caught me. He pulled out his blade. I pulled out mine. I was faster. I went up on manslaughter... They never caught on...thought I was in the henhouse trying to steal their stags... It took time—refining, inbreeding, cross-breeding, brother to sister, mother to son, adding power, rapid attack...but I think we got him.

(Gallo stands still for a beat, checks his watch, takes off his jacket and faces center stage. A slow, howling drumbeat begins. As it gradually goes higher in pitch and excitement mounts, we see narrow beams of light, the first light of dawn, filtering through the chicken wire. The light reveals a heap of chicken feathers which turns out to be an actor/dancer who represents the rooster Zapata.

90

ROOSTERS

Zapata stretches his wings, then his neck, to greet the light. *He*
stands and struts proudly, puffs his chest and crows his salutation to
the sun. *Gallo stalks Zapata, as drums follow their movements.)*
Ya, ya, mi lindo...yeah, baby...you're a beauty, a real beauty.
Now let's see whatcha got. *(He pulls out a switchblade stiletto.* *It*
gleams in the light as he tosses it from hand to hand) Come on baby
boy. Show Daddy whatcha got.
(Gallo lunges at Zapata. The rooster parries with his beak and
wings. *This becomes a slow, rhythmic fight-dance, which continues*
until Gallo grabs Zapata by his comb, bending his head backwards
until he is forced to sit. *Gallo stands behind Zapata, straddling him,*
one hand still holding the comb, the other holding the knife against
the rooster's neck.)
Oh yeah, you like to fight? Huh? You gonna kill for me baby
boy? Huh?
(Gallo sticks the tip of the knife into Zapata. *The rooster*
squawks in pain.)
Sssh! Baby boy, you gotta learn. Daddy's gotta teach you.
(Gallo sticks it to Zapata again. *This time the rooster snaps*
back in anger.)
That's right beauty... Now you got it... Come on, come.
(Gallo waves his knife and hand close to Zapata's face. The
rooster's head and eyes follow.)
Oh yeah...that's it baby, take it! Take it!
(Suddenly Zapata attacks, drawing blood. *Gallo's body*
contracts in orgasmic pleasure/pain.)
Ay precioso!... Mi lindo... You like that, eh? Taste good,
huh? *(He waves the gleaming knife in a slow hypnotic movement*
which calms the rooster.) Take my blood, honey... I'm in you
now... Morales blood, the blood of kings...and you're my rooster...
a Morales rooster. *(He slowly backs away from the rooster.* *He*
picks up his suitcase, still pointing the knife at Zapata) Kill. You're
my son. Make me proud.

ROOSTERS
by Milcha Sanchez-Scott
Southwest - Present - Hector (20's)

Hector is the son left behind when Gallo is sent to jail. This sardonic young man masks his feelings of abandonment and lonliness with satiric wit. He works as a farm laborer and here reveals contempt for his life.

HECTOR: [Nine minutes...] I will now put on the same old smelly, shit-encrusted boots, I will walk to the fields. The scent of cow dung and rotting vegetation will fill the air. I will wait with the same group of beaten-down, pathetic men...taking their last piss against a tree, dropping hard warm turds in the bushes. All adding to this fertile whore of a valley. At 7:30 that yellow mechanical grasshopper, the Deerfield tractor, will belch and move. At this exact moment, our foreman, John Knipe, will open his pig-sucking mouth, exposing his yellow, pointy, plaque-infested teeth. He yells, "Start picking, boys." The daily war begins...the intimidation of violent growth...the expanding melons and squashes, the hardiness of potatoes, the waxy purple succulence of eggplant, the potency of ripening tomatoes. All so smug, so rich, so ready to burst with sheer generosity and exuberance. They mock me... I hear them... "Hey Hector," they say, "show us whatcha got," and "Yo Hector we got bacteria out here more productive than you."... I look to the ground. Slugs, snails, worms slithering in the earth with such ferocious hunger they devour their own tails, flies oozing out larvae, aphids, bees, gnats, caterpillars their prolification only slightly dampened by our sprays. We still find eggsacks hiding, ready to burst forth. Their teeming life, their lust, is shameful...a mockery of me and my slender spirit... Well it's time... Bye Ma.

SAN ANTONIO SUNSET
by Willy Holtzman
San Antonio, TX - 1936-38 - Stone (30)

Stone has traveled all the way to San Antonio in search of Johnson, a blues guitar player whom he hopes to sign in a recording contract. Here, Stone reveals his fatigue with life on the road.

STONE: I'm not looking. I'm not looking for shit. Put two dollars together. And two more to that. And make the dollars add up to a day. A day to a week to a month to a year. And more than that, I do not know. Do not want to know. *(A beat)* I was in Philadelphia. No place to be. A place to do. Business. I do my business, and I'm looking at the road. The road—I don't have to tell you—it gets to where it's looking back. And about this time you get thirsty. Find a joint. Rough joint? Who gives a shit? The rougher the better. You only want a few. And, fuck it, you close the place. *(A beat)*

And the weather...is...hot. Not Texas hot, but hot enough. The type of weather where dogs fall over on the street; the neighbor comes at you with a bread knife. What I mean to say is—no buck-a-throw sweatbox fleabag tonight. No, sir. Got to be moving. Get the air running past you. Push the poison through the pores. Moving...to...music. But the radio, weather like that...the radio finds things...things you didn't set out to find. *(A beat)*

And that night, the radio...how do you figure?...the radio waves had to be jumping like a june bug...because, because I'm in the car, on the road, and I'm doing the knobs, looking for my music. Something out of New York. And Jesus Christ, next thing I know, I'm listening to a station in Mississippi, a place so small, I never heard, and I've been to the smallest...and, what am I hearing? What am I hearing? Because my hands on the damn know...and what's coming out...my hand just falls away...because the music coming out, it's washing over me like the hot night air. I'm...surrounded... filled with it. *(A beat)*

93

SAN ANTONIO SUNSET

And what comes at me...right at me...right between the goddamn eyes is...slide guitar. Ride hard on the high notes. Tickle the lows with the thumb. And the voice...like nothing I ever heard before...like somebody big had ahold of him. *(A beat)*

Like somebody big had a hold of you. *(A beat)*

What was I thinking? I never should've come back. What was I thinking? Crossing over.

SAN ANTONIO SUNSET
by Willy Holtzman
San Antonio, TX - 1936-38 - Johnson (20's)

Here, the young bluesman reveals uncanny insight into the
nature of the human soul as he explains his vision of God to
Stone.

JOHNSON: It's all that blackness, ain't it? Oh, the devil, he's a
craft one. Get folks to thinkin' soul's a white thing, all air and
alabaster. But we know better, you and me. We know that's how
the devil holds on to folks—get them to thinkin' they movin' closer
to heaven, when all they doin' is stayin' bodily longer. Get folks to
lookin' up find God, when all the time God's right here under foot.
(Stomps the floor)
    But you and me, Mr. Stone, we know better. It's all that
blackness. All my days, been told it's a' ugly thing, a whippin'
thing, a hatin' thing, a hangin' thing, till it sends you inside
yourself. Deep inside. And what you find, well, black ain't the
color o' hate. Black the color of the soul. You, me, ever'body.
You, Mr. Stone, it's a black piece. Hid. Hid real good. But not
so good you didn't find it. And find it again. First bad. Then
good. And, good Lord, with me, it's a little closer to the surface.
The skin itself. All that blackness. Sometimes think if I was to
prick my finger, soul'd come runnin' out the hole, so close it's to
the surface. *(Pause.)*
    All that blackness. The soul itself. And it passes out, don't
need no body no more, it don't float up like a damn balloon. Hell
no—that's the devil's foolery. No sir. The soul runs into the earth.
The black earth. 'Cause that's where God is. That's where heaven
is. Why there's more heaven in one lump of mud than in a mile of
sky. But we know that, you and me.

A SHAYNA MAIDEL
by Barbara Lebow
Brooklyn - 1946 - Mordechai Weiss (60-70)

Mordechai Weiss is the patriarch of a family of Polish jews who was fortunate enough to have emigrated to New York before the war with his daughter, Rose. His wife and older daughter stayed behind, only to be swept into the whirlwind of war and swallowed up in the camps. Shortly after the war, Lusia, the older daughter who has survived the camps, makes her way to Brooklyn. Here, Mordechai encourages her to learn to adapt to her new life as quickly as possible.

MORDECHAI: Ninety-five, ninety-six, ninety-seven, ninety-eight— [ROSE: Papa!]
MORDECHAI: *(Waving Rose off, not losing a beat.)* Sha! Ninety-nine, one hundred! *(Mordechai stops, breathes deeply, as if taking a bow, talks to Lusia, who only nods in response.)* Look. You see? I'm breathing like a teenager. In two months I'll be seventy. Also is teaching you how to count American. *(To Rose.)* I want she should know what a strong family she comes from. *(Mordechai turns back to Lusia, while Rose finishes tidying the dinette.)* Mine grandfather lived to a hundred two, still walking every day with a milk-wagon three miles. And he never missed in his life even one Sabbath in the *shul*. Finally, he died *fun* a frostbite that turned green. As it happened, he got frozen in the snow, with the milk coming up *fun* the cans, on Monday. He died just in time before sunset Friday and that's the first one he missed. This story I heard *fun* mine own mother, may she rest in peace, many times as a boy. So you know you're *fun* strong people. *(To Rose.)* You, too. Both of you. Even when I was born, on that same night, came soldiers on horses, cossacks, making trouble, setting fires. But I didn't cry and call attention. I didn't make even a peep.
[ROSE: *(Coming over and sitting.)* Papa, you told me this before, didn't you? When I was little. I never heard you tell a story since then.]

A SHAYNA MAIDEL

[MORDECHAI: So now you heard.]

[ROSE: *(Enthusiastically.)* Tell another, Papa. From when you were a boy, about your family. We'd both like to hear it. Lusia?]

[*(Lusia nods.)*]

MORDECHAI: *(Abruptly, to Rose.)* Stories should only mean something. They should teach something, like Torah. If it's not teaching something, it's a waste of time to talk so much! I want she should know also how much respect this family got. *(To Lusia.)* English. Now, Greenspan's an old man. Only seventy-two, but already an old man and I'm running the place. He, Greenspan, he calls me Morty, but no one else. Customers, salesgirls, everyone, "Good morning, Mr. Weiss" and "Let me speak to Mr. Weiss, he knows the answer." Look, I got even a business card. You see that? Mordechai Weiss. You understand? It's important you should know this. No matter how much you suffer, what you lose your family, you don't hardly know no English, you still can be a person with respect, which is worth more than all the tea in China. You understand? Your sister, she got it easier. American all the way. Nobody's gonna give her no trouble. You see that?

[ROSE: Papa, I've had to work hard, too, and—]

MORDECHAI: You got brains and health, that's what you're supposed to do! So don't tell me.

[ROSE: I know it's not the same, but I never had anyone to help me with—]

MORDECHAI: *(Hitting the floor with his cane.)* Tuchter! Mit God's *hilf*, you got brains and health you help yourself! This way you can live through anything. *(To Lusia.)* All right, *tuchter*. Get your hat and coat. We're going. *(He puts on his hat and stands up, ready to leave.)*

T BONE N WEASEL
Jon Klein
South Carolina - Present - T-Bone (30's)

T-Bone is a small-time car thief travelling the backroads of
South Carolina with his friend, Weasel. When Weasel is taken
in by a scheming politician, T-Bone steals another car and winds
up in a jail cell that he shares with a preacher, who he wastes no
time in setting straight.

T-BONE: No I dont wanna cigarette I wanna know why you
preachers gotta assume ever body lying in a jail cell caint wait to
feast they eyes on a man o the cloth. This gonna be hard fer you to
unnerstan but I dont want you. I want a woman. Git me a woman
or ask God to send me one. While you at it tell him I want a few
answers to some questions disturbin my mind. Sech as if God be so
disgusted with the human race that he set up places like this why dint
he just wipe us all out with the Flood in the first place. Or is it all
some kinda game with him like the one he played with Abraham.
Some angel come down an tell me to sacrifice *my* son I whip that
angels ass. An Job what a sorry son of a bitch standin round thankin
God ever time he gits kicked in the nuts. I wont put up with that
shit an you can go tell that to God. An where the hell did Jesus go,
up there watchin the dog races ever day whens he plannin to come
back anyway. Maybe he jest plain *forgot*. An whats God got to
offer a feller like me? He gonna stick me in some place where all
I do is sit around worshippin *him?* Got news fer you Brother Tim
that might be *yore* idea of eternal bliss but it jest dont cut it with me.
Tell you something else. I see them pictures o God when I was in
school an the cat is *white*. So what you got to say Brother Tim I be
all ears lay the Word on me.

TROUT
by William R. Lewis
Up a creek - Bert (50's)

Bert and his long-time friend, Charlie are trout fishing on a mountain stream. As the two old buddies banter about everything from aesthetics to Gandhi, trout come and go. Here, the pragmatic Bert lectures on the difference between hunting and fishing.

BERT: Hmmmm. Gandhi. *(Long pause)* I used to hunt. My father taught me. He was quite a hunter, my father. Birds, mostly. Oh, he fished, too. But he was in the main a hunter. Of course, fishing is a form of hunting. Fishing is a form of hunting, but not hunting in the strict sense. There are two reasons why this is true. Firstly, the hunter seeks his prey on the prey's own ground and in a sporting manner suitable to the prey's own rules of the game. The angler, on the other hand, does not enter the water with the fish, that is to say that although the angler might be *in* the water, he is not *under* the water...under the surface of the water...with his prey. So, a whole new set of rules apply. Secondly, the hunter has one ultimate goal: to find his prey and kill it. There is no doubt about the fact that the prey comes up short in that regard. The angler will, upon capturing his prey, have the choice of killing it or releasing it. Setting it free in the water to live. To breathe through its gills, to reproduce, to eat and grow and thrive. Or at least to be captured by a less charitable angler or another larger creature further up on the old food chain. Knowing that simple fact, being aware of it, no matter how subtly, makes the angler smug. Are there questions?

TROUT
by William R. Lewis
Up a creek - Charlie (50's)

In a moment of self-induced revelation, Charlie tells Bert of his mission in life.

CHARLIE: After Sandra passed away, I drank quite a bit. Far too much for far too long. I finally realized that I was supposed to live, not to die. Not to join my wife in whatever great or narrow water lies upstream. Then, I came to realize one other thing. That to fish, to be an angler, a true angler, was to be a kind of priest. I am a shepherd of the water. My soul flows and ebbs and moves in this impermeable current that is, in fact, my self. I am not a fisher of men, for that is what I was taught when I was a boy. Now, I am a man, and I am obligated to throw away many of the things I learned when I was young. Fishers of men have built-in excuses for pulling in empty nets. And they have precious little free time for real fishing. No, I am an angler. The highest form of life above the water. And practicing my craft keeps me keenly aware of my responsibilities. I am a piscatorial nimrod! A magician, a scorcerer and conjurer of images on flowing water wherein dwells my sober soul. I am shaman, Bertie! This bamboo wand is my pen, my staff, and my sword! I exist, by God. I am, Bertie, A FISHERMAN!!!!!

TROUT
by William R. Lewis
Up a creek - Charlie (50's)

As the sun sets, Charlie tells Bert of a near-mystical experience
he once had while fishing.

CHARLIE: Let me tell you a story. This really happened. Once,
I was fishing a lake in the high mountains. A small lake. More of
a pond, really. The water was very cold. And the sky and the
mountains were reflected on the surface. Often it was very difficult
to tell which was water and which was sky. I had been fishing all
day, and the sun was about to set. The sky was red, and the air was
taking on the chill of evening. A flock of geese, their silhouettes
honking and streaming, passed overhead, heading for structure. I
was drinking whiskey—ancient autumnal, peat-inspired whiskey. It
was whiskey season. Whiskey seasons were longer then. I was
fishing with a Clark Special, which hung on the surface like a small
chunk of a leftover dream. Sandra had recently gone to her reward
and I was feeling very blue. I spent a lot of time drinking and
fishing, and crying. Often, all at the same time. But this time was
different. Different and very special. The Clark Special would sail
off through the crisp, thin air and land so gently on the water.
Check cast. Wait. Count. Strip. Count. Strip. And so on.
Then, without my totally noticing, the water began to show me
things. People I hadn't seen in years. Sounds I hadn't heard. I saw
Sandra on the still, glassy surface. In it. On it. Like a living
person reflected in the water, but there was nothing to reflect. She
smiled at me. She asked if they were biting, and if I wanted to eat
dinner at home or to go out for a late supper. I saw myself as a
young boy, helping my grandfather lay a fire in his fireplace. His
hands would touch my small shoulders. He laughed and lit his pipe.
I struck a match and my grandfather heaped on kindling. He peeled
an apple for me with his pocketknife, and the sweet juice dribbled
from my chin as I munched apples, and smelled my grandfather's
pipe. I saw Sandra again, this time as a young bride who depended

TROUT

far too much on her stripling groom. She was very serious then. And I saw my father, sitting at another fireplace, doing what he did best in all the world. Holding the knife he had inherited from his father in his nimble, brown hands. He created flyrods. Split bamboo. White birch. Curls of wood piled at his feet by the fire. Once, and I saw this too—in the water of that lake in the mountains—my father was stripping the bark from a long branch that was too be my own first flyrod. The knife slipped off the wood and dug into the fleshy web of my father's gentle hand. Blood spurted and ran from the wound. But my father only held his hands together, folded as if in prayer, and he stared into the fire and smiled. All of this, I saw on the surface of a lake in the mountains of America. And, as the vision vanished, I snapped the Clark Special back off the surface in preparation for another cast, and... and blood dripped from the fly. And I was not afraid.

THE WOMAN IN BLACK
adapted by Stephen Mallatratt
from the book by Susan Hill
A London Theatre - Kipps (30-40)

Arthur Kipps is a man who is literally haunted by the past. In an effort to free himself from visitations from "the Woman in Black", a spectre who has attached herself to Kipps in order to avenge the death of her young child, Kipps hires out a theater and an actor and proceeds to reenact his first meeting with the phantom. His ghostly tale begins on Christmas Eve...

KIPPS: *(reading)* It was nine-thirty on Christmas Eve. As I opened my front door and stepped outside I smelled at once, and with a lightening heart, that there had been a change in the weather. All the previous week we had had thin chilling rain and a mist that lay low about the house and over the countryside. My spirits have for many years been excessively affected by the weather. But now the dampness and fogs had stolen away like thieves into the night, the sky was pricked over with stars and the full moon rimmed with a halo of frost. Upstairs, three children slept with stockings tied to their bedposts. There was something in the air that night. That my peace of mind was about to be disturbed, and memories awakened that I had thought for ever dead, I had, naturally, no idea. That I should ever again renew my acquaintance with mortal dread and terror of spirit, would have seemed at that moment impossible. I took a last look at the frosty darkness, sighed contentedly, and went in, to the happy company of my family. At the far end of the room stood the tree, candlelit and bedecked, and beneath it were the presents. There were vases of white chrysanthemums, and in the centre of the room a pyramid of gilded fruit and a bowl of oranges stuck all about with cloves, their spicy scent filling the air and mingling with the wood-smoke to be the very aroma of Christmas. I became aware that I had interrupted the others in a lively conversation. "We are telling ghost stories—just the thing for Christmas Eve!" And so they were—vying with each other to tell

103

the horridest, most spine-chilling tale. They told of dripping stone walls in uninhabited castles and of ivy-clad monastery ruins by moonlight, of locked inner rooms and secret dungeons, dark charnel houses and overgrown graveyards, of howlings and shriekings, groanings and scuttlings. This was a sport, a high-spirited and harmless game among young people, there was nothing to torment and trouble me, nothing of which I could possibly disapprove. I did not want to seem a killjoy, old, stodgy and unimaginative. I turned my head away so that none of them should see my discomfiture. "And now it's your turn." "Oh no," I said, "nothing for me." "You must know at least one ghost story, everyone knows *one*." Ah, yes, yes, indeed. All the time I had been listening to their ghoulish, lurid inventions, the one thought that had been in my mind, and the only thing I could have said was "No, no, you have none of you any idea. This is all nonsense, fantasy, it is not like this. Nothing so blood-curdling and becreepered and crude—not so...so laughable. The truth is quite other, and altogether more terrible. I am sorry to disappoint you," I said. "But I have no story to tell!" And went quickly from the room and from the house. I walked in a frenzy of agitation, my heart pounding, my breathing short. I had always known in my heart that the experience would never leave me, that it was woven into my very fibres. Yes, I had a story, a true story, a story of haunting and evil, fear and confusion, horror and tragedy. But it was not a story to be told around the fireside on Christmas Eve.

AWAY
by Michael Gow
Australia - Christmas, 1967 - Jim (40's)

Jim's marriage to the shrewish Gwen has become more and more like a nightmare with each passing day. It was not always so, and here he tells his daughter of how different Gwen was when they were courting.

JIM: When we were first courting I took her to the pictures to see *Gone With the Wind*. Afterwards she was so quiet, but excited, something in her head was turning over and over. She was living in this funny little house in Surry Hills then, with all her sisters, it was a pretty dirty area. The next week I went round to take her out to a dance.

Everyone else had gone on some church picnic and she was home on her own so I knew we'd have a few minutes alone. I got there a bit early because I couldn't think of anything else I'd rather be doing. I went round the back and as I went past the kitchen window I could hear her talking to someone. I stopped at the back door. She was saying what old Vivien Leigh said in *Gone With the Wind*—just before the intermission and the war's been on and everyone's dead and the house's wrecked and the crops burnt and she's scratching around in the dirt for some old potato or cotton or something just to feed her family and she stands up against that red sky and says: 'As God is my witness, I will never be hungry again.' I laughed, not at her but I was really bowled over, she was as good as old Vivien any day. She was very embarrassed and so was I and we made a bit of a joke of it. But seeing her upset before made me remember that afternoon. 'I will never be hungry again.' It had that effect on a lot of people, that film. Old Scarlet standing in that field and wanting to rule the world.

AWAY
by Michael Gow
Australia - Christmas, 1967 - Harry (40's)

Harry's son is dying of cancer. The family has recently moved from England to Australia and now they find themselves celebrating Christmas on the beach with new friends. Here, Harry tells Jim about his son's illness.

HARRY: This is a wonderful country. We're still not used to a hot Christmas.

[JIM: My wife is not really an angry woman. She has high hopes.]

HARRY: We have no regrets. We don't get homesick. Only once a year. We book a telephone call to our old street. In Nottingham. We get out the photo album. Remember for a while. But we have no regrets. This country...and often when we do think back, all we can think of is the cold, the tiny houses, the rationing, the rubble after the war. It was a rubbish dump. A lot wanted to stay and help to build again. But we didn't want to. We felt held back. We knew why the sailors had called it the Old World. It was like living with an elderly relative, tired, cranky, who doesn't want you to have any fun but just worry about their health all the time. Nagging you, criticising you, making you feel guilty for any enjoyment you might manage to find. No regrets. In a funny kind of way we're happy. Even while we're very, very sad. We have no regrets, but we have no hopes. Not any more. We might get some, but it's unlikely, I think. Our son is very sick. It's a cancer of the blood. He was very bad this year, we thought it was time to get ready. But he got through it. It's called 'in remission'. But it will come back. Every day we watch for bruises. Or to see if he's more tired than usual. We made it into another year at least. But we don't look forward. We haven't given up, no, no. That would be a mistake. We don't look back and we don't look forward. We have this boy and we won't have him for long. And whatever he does, that will have to be enough. The Chinese don't believe in being too upset when someone dies. That would mean you thought they'd died too soon and what they'd done up till then didn't amount to much. We will be sad, of course.

GOOSE AND TOMTOM
by David Rabe
Underworld apartment - Recently - Goose (20-30)

Goose and Tomtom are jewel theives whose souls struggle for
survival in a purgatory-like setting where they seem condemmed
to commiting acts of violence. During his journey from life to
this surrealisitic place, Goose has been given insight into his true
nature as he here reveals to Tomtom.

GOOSE: I mean, it was before I lived around here. I don't know
where it was, but I was in this room, and I couldn't get out. But I
don't give a fuck. It's happened before. And then, all of a sudden,
there's all this dark behind me that's different than all the other dark,
and in this different dark, there is the reason that it's different, and
the reason is it's a ghost behind me, and when I turn to look he just
moves so he stays behind me, and then he says like into the back of
my head, "Don't you wanna know the secret?" And I say, "No, I
don't." An' he says, "It's a secret about you, don't you wanna
know it?" And I say, "No," an' I'm wishin' he would go away, and
he hears my thinkin', so he's angry.
(Tomtom spasms, getting sicker, and Goose goes to the downstage
crates from which Tomtom got the aspirins. Goose gets a
thermometer, a stethoscope, aspirin, perhaps something for the pins.
Going back to Tomtom, he tends him.)
GOOSE: All of a sudden in his anger I can't move anymore, and
then I can, but I can't stand up, or talk. And all of a sudden I know
why all the other little kids in the neighborhood hate me, 'cause they
do, and tease me, 'cause they do, and it's 'cause I'm a frog. 'At's
the secret about me. And now he's brought it up outa the secret
places in me and into my body; this ghost with these eyes has looked
at me an' turned me into a frog in me. *(Pause.)* Well, I'm cryin'—
I'm not afraid to tell you, Tomtom, I'm cryin' an' beggin', I'll do
anything he wants—I don't know what it is—but I can't move or
speak, all green and spotty. So the night is on and on, and it's truer
than anything else. I belong on my belly. Out of doors an' wet and

cold. Out by green scummy ponds unable to talk all my feelin's or thoughts but burstin' with 'em. Layin' inna wet slimy grass, hopin' to lick some fly outa the air. Worms around me an' spiders. The night seems so long. As years an' years. And then there's light, an' I see my body's a person again, 'cause I made the ghost a promise I don't know what it was. *(Slight pause.)* An' sometimes, I still get feelings of a frog an' I gotta look around and check everything real good an' make sure I'm not layin' in green wet grass wantin' to eat flies, 'cause I'm cold in my heart sometimes. I'm all spotty an' green in my heart. In my heart I know where I belong, an' I got big buggy eyes. *(Pause.)* That fuckin' promise to a ghost, I made it—I don't know what it was, but I know I'm keepin' it. He said I would be a frog as long as he was a ghost, and blood was red and mud wet an' secrets secrets. You ever made a promise to a ghost? Tom... tom?

GOOSE AND TOMTOM
by David Rabe
Underworld apartment - Recently - Bingo (30's)

Tomtom and Goose have kidnapped Bingo's sister, Lulu, in an
effort to recover diamonds which they believe were stolen from
them by Bingo. Wandering through the underworld in search of
his beloved Lulu, Bingo finally arrives at the home of Tomtom
and Goose, where he tells his tale.

BINGO *(continuing)*: I am being punished and I deserve it, but I
can't stand it. I expected some other punishment, to be shot or
maimed. But not to lose my sister and feel so lost. We was making
plans for our future. Certain changes were going to be made. I
heard a noise, a sort of half a scream, but I however paid no
attention. I was deep in thought and worry, knowing how I did how
I was going to be punished. I knew people everywhere was angry
at me because I been poor and I been mean, so I done dirt. But I
got a right to my own sister. We would hug. We would pet. I
could whirl her by the legs and she would howl. It made me feel
good. I know I got reasons for which I can be punished. I blown
people away. I'm a action guy, whatas anybody want? I done
dynamite and sealed away many a problem and got away clean,
'cause I know who was who from the day I showed up— So I
buried many a person out in the marshes so his guts are huggin' the
roots a flowers and he's eye to eye with many a dead rat, but I still
got a right to see my own sister. I can't live without her. I lied.
I lied. There was scarcely any intervening time between my sister's
arrival here and my own. We were twins. We were planning a
walk in the woods, holding hands. I could look into her face and see
my own. And then I came out of that room and she was gone. It
was as if a terrible wind had blown through that room and taken her.
I called her name. I could hear the wind receding. In the hallway,
I found an old woman, a hag of a woman, and she was smoking a
pipe and smiling. She looked in the direction my sister had gone,
and I followed her glance. I been on the street. I followed a trail

of old roses and bits of clothing. Paper bags. Debris arranged in a cryptic manner. I've been alone. I saw your light. I couldn't bear it anymore. I needed human voices. I needed to tell my story. I waited for daybreak. I had a premonition there would be trouble. No one came or went. I waited. I knocked. You let me in. You tied me up.

KVETCH
by Stephen Berkoff
Frank and Donna's house - Present - Hal (30-40)

Hal is recently divorced and still somewhat reluctant to socialize. When Frank, a co-worker, invites him home for dinner, he accepts and finds that he actually enjoys being out after so many months of solitary existence in his lonely apartment. Here are Hal's ruminations as the evening progresses.

HAL: *This is really a nice family...warm-hearted...kind... How nice of him to ask me... See, I'm warming up... I feel OK again... Maybe one day I'll have them over to me... Yeah, I'll make dinner for them...but I'm not a good cook... Oh, no, I've got the demons coming on...go away, go away!! I was happy before... Go away!... I can't be invited here again and not reciprocate... They maybe don't expect it but how many times can I be invited before reciprocating? Once...twice...three times?... I could make something simple and we'll have a few drinks... We'll eat in the kitchen and then go in the living room for coffee... Must I think of it now?... I'll make some snacks...just a little soupcon of every- thing... I'll get it from the deli and then we'll have it in the living room... Should we start in the living room with drinks then go to the kitchen?... But if I'm preparing something hot, say a soup, I'll have to leave them in the living room with a drink and run in and out... or...why not start off in the kitchen with drinks?... But then the stereo is in the living room... Oh, shit...we can play some music and have a few drinks and then go into the kitchen...or still better... I'll leave them a drink and bring the stuff into the living room... But why shlapp it in the living room when the kitchen is supposed to be where you dine?... Unless I bring the stereo into the kitchen... but what if we go after to the living room for coffee?... I can't shlapp it back again... Maybe I'll buy another cassette deck... No, I'll put all the stuff in the living room and run in and out and most of the stuff will be cold anyway, except for the soup and the coffee... Mind you, it's cosy in the kitchen... There's a big wooden table in there...*

111

KVETCH

In the living room there's small tables so I'll have to take the salad round...to where people are sitting at the small tables... There's no centre table so we couldn't all face each other with a bottle in the middle... I'll have to walk around with the bottle...but at least there'll be space...but it won't be so warm as the kitchen... Oh, fuck it, we'll eat in there...that's fine...take the consequences... But it would be nice for them to see the living room...after, with coffee...not before...no after...not before? Wait!... We could eat in the living room if I brought the table into the centre, then I could put the bottle in the middle... That means taking the table from the kitchen...but then after we've eaten we'll have to sit in the living room with all the dirty dishes or make a fuss clearing them up whereas in the kitchen you just leave it all and say, let's stretch our feet in the living room... No, I know what to do... I'll kill myself instead...then I won't have to do anything...take an overdose or get run down by a truck... This is why God breathed life into me...to decide whether the table goes in the living room or in the kitchen...oooohh!

KVETCH
by Stephen Berkoff

Frank and Donna's house - Present - Frank (30-40)
Frank is the blustery host of the impromptu dinner party. As he
tells a joke, he relfects with pride on his ability to amuse and
then realizes with horror that he is boring everyone.

FRANK: So he's sitting in the movie house and thinks, 'So vy not
see it again'... *Gosh, this is going really well... I'm excited...
Hey, I can easily hold them there in the palm of my hand... I knew
I could do it, so why do I hold back, why lack confidence when I'm
such a marvellous story-teller?... I have the power... I know I do...
but I always let the others do it...let them be funny...take the
stage...impress the ladies and I go quiet and choke and then I open
my mouth with a prepared speech and it sounds like death 'cause it
didn't come out when it went in my head... I let it spoil and then
when I let it out it stinks like day-old herring you forgot to put back
in the fridge... Oh, God, the joke's a prepared speech so what am
I talking about? Yeah, but it's different, you got to use timing. Now
timing's the gold of the comic...without timing, a shitty story will
come across like a shitty story. But with timing a shitty story will
sound like poetry...no, not poetry...but like amazing...like brilliant...
A golden observation...but a brilliant observation will sound like a
drek in the mouth of a shmock! You know...don't laugh, but maybe
I could do cabaret... Yeah, get up on volunteer nights in the bar
down the street... 'Hey, ladies and gentlemen, what's a Jewish
American princess's favourite wine?'... Gentiles love Jewish jokes...
I could get up and tell a lot of anti-Semitic jokes and I could get
away with it... Oh, I know a beauty... I'll save it for after this...*
Yeah, vy not indeed...so he sees the film again, he likes it so much
that he stays for the last show... *Why are they yawning?... No, it's
not going down too well...it's terrible...I promise God I won't tell
anti-Semitic jokes... Just let me get to the end...please... I wish I
never started... Why do I want to be funny and tell jokes?... I hate
telling jokes... I hate it... I can't tell jokes... I'll never be able to
tell them... I've never told them so why did I insist?... I loathe it...
I'm going hot and cold...why on earth do I give myself this
torture?...*

113

LARGO DESOLATO
by Vaclav Havel
English version by Tom Stoppard
Leopold's living room - Present - Leopold (40's)

Professor Leopold Nettles has written a book which contains a paragraph considered offensive by the repressive government under which he lives. As menacing, shadowy figures begin appearing at his door to pressure him to sign a document which disavows his work, Nettles feels as though he has lost control of his life. Here, he confesses his despair to his lover.

LEOPOLD: I feel sorry for you, Lucy—
[LUCY: Why?]
LEOPOLD: You deserve someone better. I'm just worthless—
[LUCY: I don't like you talking about yourself like that—]
LEOPOLD: It's true, Lucy. I can't get rid of the awful feeling that lately something has begun to collapse inside me—as if some axis which was holding me together has broken, the ground collapsing under my feet, as if I'd gone lame inside—I sometimes have the feeling that I'm acting the part of myself instead of being myself. I'm lacking a fixed point out of which I can grow and develop. I'm erratic—I'm letting myself be tossed about by chance currents—I'm sinking deeper and deeper into a void and I can no longer get a grip on things. In truth I'm just waiting for this thing that's going to happen and am no longer the self-aware subject of my own life but becoming merely its passive object—I have a feeling sometimes that all I am doing is listening helplessly to the passing of the time. What happened to my perspective on things? My humour? My industry and persistence? The pointedness of my observations? My irony and self-irony? My capacity for enthusiasm, for emotional involvement, for commitment, even for sacrifice? The oppressive atmosphere in which I have been forced to live for so long is bound to have left its mark! Outwardly I go on acting my role as if nothing has happened but inside I'm no longer the person you all take me for. It's hard to admit it to myself, but if *I* can all the more reason

114

for you to! It's a touching and beautiful thing that you don't lose hope of making me into someone better than I am but—don't be angry—it's an illusion. I've fallen apart, I'm paralysed, I won't change and it would be best if they came for me and took me where I would no longer be the cause of unhappiness and disillusion—

THE GOLDEN AGE
by Louis Nowra
Tasmania - 1935-1945 - Francis (20-30)

When Francis and his friend, Peter, go camping in the wilds of
Tasmania, they stumble upon the survivors of a shipwrecked
group of convicts who have been living in a feral state since the
Victorian age. Francis becomes attracted to Betsheb, a member
of the strange tribe with a captivating lust for life. Although she
doesn't understand English, Francis tells her about his world.

FRANCIS: Are you looking at the sunset?
(Startled, BETSHEB turns around.)
(Smiling) I'm not a monster... No more running.
(Silence. He walks closer to the river.)
Look at us reflected in the water, see? Upside-down.
(He smiles and she smiles back. Silence.)
So quiet. I'm not used to such silence. I'm a city boy, born and
bred. You've never seen a city or town, have you? Where I live
there are dozens of factories: shoe factories, some that make gaskets,
hydraulic machines, clothing. My mother works in a shoe factory.
(Pointing to his boots) These came from my mother's factory.
(Silence.)
These sunsets here, I've never seen the likes of them. A bit of
muddy orange light in the distance, behind the chimneys, is
generally all I get to see.
(Pause.)
You'd like the trams, especially at night. They rattle and squeak,
like ghosts rattling their chains, and every so often the conducting
rod hits a terminus and there is a brilliant spark of electricity, like
an axe striking a rock. 'Spisss!' On Saturday afternoon thousands
of people go and watch the football. A huge oval of grass. *(Miming
a football)* A ball like this. Someone hand passes it, 'whish',
straight to me. I duck one lumbering giant, spin around a nifty
dwarf of a rover, then I catch sight of the goals. I boot a seventy-
yard drop kick straight through the centre. The crowd goes wild!

116

THE GOLDEN AGE

(He cheers wildly. BETSHEB laughs at his actions. He is pleased to have made her laugh.)
Not as good as your play.
(Pause.)
This is your home. My home is across the water, Bass Strait.
(Silence. STEF rolls over and ends up near FRANCIS' feet.)
What is it about you people? Why are you like you are?
(BETSHEB gathers up her flowers. As she stands she drops a few.)
Don't go.
(He picks up the fallen flowers.)
I was watching you pick these. My mother steals flowers from her neighbour's front garden so every morning she can have fresh flowers in her vase for Saint Teresa's portrait. She was a woman of centuries ago. God fired a burning arrow of love into her. *(Smiling)* When it penetrated her, Saint Teresa could smell the burning flesh of her heart.

THE GRACE OF MARY TRAVERSE
by Timberlake Wertenbaker
London - 18th Century - Lord Gordon (20-30)

Lord Gordon is a man suffering the effects of his ordinary appearance and demeanor. Here, he complains bitterly of his unnoticability.

LORD GORDON: My name is George Gordon. Lord Gordon. *(Pause.)* Nothing. No reaction. No one's interested. *(Pause.)* It's always like this. I greet people, their eyes glaze. I ride in Hyde Park, my horse falls asleep. *(Pause.)* I am a man of stunning mediocrity. *(Pause.)* This can't go on. I must do something. Now. But what? How does Mr Manners make everyone turn around? Of course: politics. I'll make a speech in the House: all criminals must be severely punished. But stealing a handkerchief is already a hanging matter. I know: make England thrifty, enclose the common land. I think that's been done. Starve the poor to death! Perhaps politics is too ambitious. I'll write. Even women do that now. But about what? No, I'll be a wit. I'll make everyone laugh at what I say. But I'll have to think of something funny. Sir John's a rake, that's a possibility. But the ladies are so demanding and my manhood won't rise above middling. Shall I die in a duel? No. This is desperate. Perhaps I'm seen with the wrong people. They're all so brilliant. In a different world, I might shine. Here are some ordinary people. They must notice me, if only because I'm a lord. Oh God, please make me noticed, just once. Please show me the way.

THE GRACE OF MARY TRAVERSE
by Timberlake Wertenbaker
London - 18th Century - Mr. Hardlong (30-40)

Mary Traverse has run away from her wealthy father in order to experience life before resigning herself to marriage with a man she doesn't love. She had paid Mr. Hardlong to have sex with her. When she hesitates to join him in bed, he encourages her with the following words.

MR HARDLONG: You ask for pleasure. Why do you cringe as if expecting violence?
(Short silence.)
If you believe violence will bring you pleasure, you've been misled. The enjoyment of perversion is not a physical act but a metaphysical one. You want a pleasure: come and take it.
(Silence. MARY does not move.)
Are you pretending you've never felt desire unfurl in your blood? Never known the gnawing of flesh, that gaping hunger of the body? Never sensed the warm dribble of your longings? Come, come, need isn't dainty and it's no good calling cowardice virginity.
(MARY squirms a little.)
Perhaps you want me to seduce you and let you remain irresponsible? I promise you physical pleasure, not the tickle of self-reproach and repentance, the squirm of the soul touching itself in its intimate parts. Or are you waiting for a declaration of love? Let romance blunt the sting of your need, mask a selfish act with selfless acquiescence? Novels, my dear, novels. And in the end, your body remains dry. What are you waiting for? Pleasure requires activity. Come.
(MARY moves a little closer and closes her eyes.)
Ah, yes. Close the eyes, let the act remain dark: Cling to your ignorance, the mind's last chastity. A man's body is beautiful, Mary, and ought to be known. I'll even give you some advice, for free: never take a man you don't find beautiful. If you have to close your eyes when he comes near you, turn away, walk out of the room

119

and never look back. You may like his words, his promises, his wit, his soul, but wrapping your legs around a man's talent will bring no fulfilment. No, open your eyes. Look at me.

(MARY looks, unfocused.)

The neck is beautiful, Mary, but doesn't require endless study. Look down. The arms have their appeal and the hands hold promise. The chest can be charming, the ribs melancholic. Look down still. They call these the loins, artists draw their vulnerability, but you're not painting a martyrdom. Look now.

(MARY focuses on his penis.)

See how delicate the skin, how sweetly it blushes at your look. It will start at your touch, obey your least guidance. It's one purpose is to serve you and you'd make it an object of fear? Look, Mary, shaped for your delight, intricacies for your play, here is the wand of your pleasure, nature's generous magic. I'm here for you. Act now. You have hands, use them. Take what you want, Mary. Take it.

LIFE AND LIMB
by Keith Reddin
USA - 1950's - Franklin (30's)

Franklin has been wounded in Korea, losing his arm in the process. When he returns to his wife, Effie, they struggle to put their lives back together. One day, Effie and a friend plan to attend a matinee at the movies and here, Franklin tells the audience of the tragic event that occured that fateful day.

FRANKLIN: Freud, in his dynamics of the personality defines the concept of reality anxiety as a painful emotional experience resulting from a perception of danger in the external world. A danger is any condition of the environment which threatens to harm the person. My favorite movie is the movie "The Bridges of Toko Ri" starring William Holden, Mickey Rooney and Grace Kelly. Also I was sexually aroused during certain sequences in "The Creature From the Black Lagoon," but I have never related this information to anyone. I noticed I was rooting for the Creature to attack this girl scientist and one scene where he is swimming under her, following her slowly while she is unaware of his presence gave me an erection. I looked around the theatre at this point in the movie and noticed that quite a few of the men in the audience had strange expressions on their faces also. Experiences that overpower one with anxiety are called "traumatic" because they reduce the person to an infantile state of helplessness. The prototype of all traumatic experiences is the birth trauma. The newly-born baby is bombarded with excessive stimulation from the world for which its fetal experience has not prepared it.

A 3-D sequel to "The Creature From the Black Lagoon" was released the next year due to the success of the orginal film, but I stayed away from that fearing what the consequences of three dimensional projection could cause me.

Effie and Doina never made it back from the movies that afternoon. The balcony of the Fox Theatre under which they were sitting enjoying a 2:30 showing of "Cattle Queen of Montana"

LIFE AND LIMB

starring Barbara Stanwyck and Ronald Reagan collapsed, killing them instantly. The surprise I had for Effie was a new television. While she and Doina were at the movies, I moved all the furniture around the apartment to find a place to set this new television. I was informed by the police of the accident at 4:35, she had been pronounced dead on arrival. I sent the TV back the next day. I didn't even plug it in.

THE MASK OF HIROSHIMA
by Ernest Ferlita
Hiroshima - 7 years after the bomb - Shinji (29)

As Japan struggles to rebuild following the devastation of the
war, Shinji and Hisa struggle to rebuild their lives. Here,
Shinji, who has been trying to convince Hisa to marry him,
reminds her of the flowers that bloomed after the bomb.

SHINJI: Hisa, remember how those crazy flowers
bloomed right after the bomb?
Out of the bones and ashes
they popped up all over the city.
Everywhere there were day lilies
and bluets and morning glories.
But it was horrible to see
because it was all such a lie,
nothing but a frenzied push
to be free of the poisoned earth.
And then winter came,
and they all fell away.
And people said nothing would grow
in these parts for seventy years.
But they were wrong.
(Goes down on his haunches)
The other day
I saw a morning glory still half asleep.
It looked very shy in the shade,
as if it'd rather not be noticed.
But then the sun came poking around,
and before I knew it
that little bit of a blossom
was looking up at me wide awake.
And do you know what it said to me?
It said, "I did not forget to bloom."
"People," I said, "will not forget to build,

to build houses and cities,
to build lives again."
(Rises)
Hisa, let me touch you.

OPERA COMIQUE
by Nagle Jackson
Paris - March 3, 1875 - Bizet (40's)

On the opening night of his opera, "Carmen", Geroges Bizet takes a moment during the overture to comment on the mentality of the audience, and his love for his music and his disdain for those who listen to it are obvious.

BIZET: ...well of course they like that, all that "dum da da ditty da da, dum da da ditty da da..." *(He is humming the rousing opening melody of the Overture.)* ...and they sort of look around at one another in the half-dark, tap their communal foot...the ladies remember—only *now*—all the equipment they need from their reticules...snap, snap; rustle, rustle...and they ask their spouses to do things for them: rearrange programs and gloves. They settle and arrange their pearls, wave at people they just finished talking to in the Grand Foyer. The men pick at their teeth. I mean, *why* did I spend all that time, hammering it out, rejecting it, finding it again, orchestrating it...my God, orchestrating it!...playing it for managers, teaching it to conductors, changing everything again, *re*-orchestrating it...why did I do all that for people who use it as background music for the interior voices of their own digestive juices?

But now it all changes. Now...just about now the big theme comes in... *(He opens the door to #5 and the Fate Motif is heard. He closes the door.)* I call it the Fate Motif, but I can't say that too loudly because they all accuse me of being a Wagnerian. What happens, you see, is that suddenly in the midst of all that "dum da da ditty da da" and that *boring* Toreador melody—which they're going to *love*—right in the middle of the overture comes: Fate. Destiny. *Death.* And it will be heard more and more, and then at the end of the opera—which they will *hate*—they'll hear it again, the theme of Fate...it will be the last music they hear as the curtain....

It's quite good, really. It's...well, here, you see: *(A large blow-up reprint of the fully orchestrated four measures from the Overture containing the first statement of the Fate Motif flies in right*

*next to Bizet. He takes a pointer from his pocket and continues to
lecture like a music professor.)*
    What you have here, you see, after the preceding A-major
cadence, is an abrupt, harmonic shift to D-minor...I mean you see
it in the strings...tremulo, you see, held *long*...two measures, then
the motif: "daaa da da de dum"; just a simple statement, really: D-
minor scale sort of rearranged in the, er...woodwinds, trumpets,
celli...actually sort of curious, that. I mean having the trumpets
double the cello line there to *cut through*... There again, they'll all
yell "Wagner! Wagner!" ...and then, you see, we re-emphasize the
key with the pizzicati in the contrabass and harp, the tymp and
horns...all very...I mean, *look* at this! All this. And to them it's
just...I mean, stockbrokers and bankers who could not even begin to
understand the technical complexities, dismiss it all as trivial!...
"What do you do?... You write music?...isn't that nice. Wish I
could diddle about all day at the pianoforte, but of course I've got
proper work to do..." I mean do they...could they...? *(He stops.
Looks around at where he is.)* What on earth am I doing? Well,
(Indicating music.) ...you see the whole thing here: "daa da da de
dum...boom, boom"...and you will hear it all through the...and then
at the end, it's very...it's the key to the whole thing, really,
it's...I'm sorry; I have sort of gone on and on...er...we don't need
this anymore. *(The music reprint flies out.)* I'll...er, I'll just go
back in and see how the First Act's going... *(He starts into box,
turns back.)* Remember: "Daa da da de dum...boom, boom."

126

OPERA COMIQUE
by Nagle Jackson
Paris - March 3, 1875 - Bizet (40's)

At the close of "Carmen", Bizet is confronted by a young woman in the corridor outside his box at the opera house. When she expresses her disappointment at the opera's ending, the composer explodes with anger.

BIZET: *You!* You are disappointed in me! You, who have the mind of a pancake, the heart of a hummingbird and the emotional sensitivity of a fencepost? You are disappointed in me...with your bracelets and earrings and petticoats and petty, boring soul, you are disappointed in me?? I have created a *thing* this evening, a work. My every waking moment has been focused on this day, on this night, on this...beautiful work...my beloved *Carmen*. And you—the primped and gussied dependent of some mindless functionary, you are disappointed in *me!* You come to me with alternative endings! I'll give you some alternative endings: Have you considered insignificance? Or a simple solitude in some bourgeois suburb? Or better yet, and far more likely, a meaningless communion with some third-rate, propertied toad? These are the endings I propose to you, dear mademoiselle, for they require no work, no imagination and no concern. Which is what you and everyone in this theatre have given me tonight. And now, Ernest, I shall take me to the streets and let the dust from this fiasco settle. Tell my wife. And tell the singers...tell my singers that I am sorry, heartily sorry. And tell them I shall never write a single note of music again.

TENT MEETING
by Larry Larson, Levi Lee and Rebecca Wackler
A house trailer - 1940's - Darrell (20-30)

Darrell is a WWII vet travelling with his evangelical father and sister. They have just kidnapped his sister's baby from a medical lab and plan to escape in their house trailer to Canada. The child is badly deformed and here, Darrell addresses the baby in its crib.

DARRELL: Yecch! Boy you sure are ugly. Hell, we'd have to hang a pork chop around your neck to get the dog to play with you. If we had a dog and you had a neck which we don't and you don't. You hear me? Of course you can't hear me. You need ears to hear. Can't see me either can you? Wait a minute, maybe that's an ear. Yeah, that could be an ear. Or maybe it's a hand. Nah! I don't see what's so special about you anyway. Where were you during the war, Jesus O. Tarbox? I didn't see you out where I was on the front lines in France, Europe, where it was freezin' cold out there in the field that we had to stuff newspapers in our uniforms to keep from freezing to death! I bet you are wondering about this medal. *(Fingers his Purple Heart)* This is called the Purple Heart, and except for the Congressional Medal of Honor, it's the best medal a person in the armed forces can get. I could've got a lot of other medals, but I wanted this one. They gave it to me for valor, bravery, courage and getting stuck with a bayonet. Oh yeah?! You want to see my war scar? *(HE raises his shirt)* There it is, right there. And that's why I'm not playing professional baseball to this day. If them krauts hadn't of stuck me, I'd still have my fastball. Which they did, and I don't. But I'm still better off than you. I got a good nickle curveball which is more than you've got. I got a spitball, which is more than you got. I got spit, which is more than you got. You couldn't throw a baseball if your life depended on it, which fortunately for you it don't. Hell, you can't even catch. You know, I bet if I was to take this baseball right here and throw it as hard as I can right in your...your...face, I'd probably kill you. I'd

128

probably splatter you all over this trailer. End all this craziness forever. No more hearin' how special you are. So maybe that's what I ought to do. Put you out of your misery. End all this craziness. Course if you really was Jesus, like Daddy says, you could stop me...you could stop this baseball in midair, or turn it into a rabbit or something. Is that what you're gonna do? Come on, Jesus O. Tarbox, what'll it be? You're the catcher, give me a sign. Curve or spitball? Just give me a sign.

THE WASH
by Philip Kan Gotanda
America - Present - Nobu Matsumoto (68)

After 40 years of marriage, Nobu's wife, Masi, leaves him to start a new life for herself. Their marriage had been an unhappy one, and Nobu inflicted much emotional abuse upon Masi, leaving her with feelings of isolation and despair. When he discovered that Masi is seeing another man, he flies into a rage, buys a rifle and goes to her apartment. By the time he arrives his passion is spent. He and Masi confront one another, but the time for anger is over.

NOBU: Where is he? *(Masi stares at the gun)*
[MASI: He went to buy the newspaper.]
NOBU *(Notices Masi watching him cautiously)*: It's not loaded. *(Pause)* At first I said, "No, no, no, I can't believe it. I can't believe it." I got so pissed off. I got my gun and drove over here. I drove around the block twenty or thirty times thinking, "I'm gonna shoot this son-of-a-bitch, I'm gonna shoot him." I drove up, rang the doorbell. No one answered. I kept ringing, ringing... I went back to the car and waited. You cheated on me. How could you do that to me? I'm a good husband! I'm a good husband, Masi... I kept seeing you two. The two of you together. I kept seeing that. It made me sick. I kept thinking, "I'm gonna shoot that son-of-a-bitch. I'm gonna shoot him. I waited in the car. It was three o'clock in the morning when I woke up. It was so cold in the car. You weren't back. I got worried I might catch a cold, and my back—you know how my back gets. I drove home, took a hot bath, and went to sleep. I've been sick in bed all week. I just wanted to show you. Both of you. That's why I brought it. Don't worry. It's not loaded. *(He cracks the shotgun and shows her that it is not loaded)* I just wanted to show both of you how it was, how I was feeling. But it's all right. You two. It's all right now.

ADVICE TO THE PLAYERS
by Bruce Bonafede
An American Theater - Robert Obosa (40's)

Based on an actual incident, this is the story of two black South African actors who are prevented from performing in an American play festival by the South African National Council. If they perform, the Council has threatened reprisals on their loved ones, if they don't perform, the South African government will order them banned. Here, a defeated Robert tells a grim tale of the time he was imprisoned in his homeland.

ROBERT: [No, Oliver. She's right. It's still up to us, no matter what she does. *(He moves close to Oliver.)*] You know, in my last year in prison I was most of the time alone. But once, for awhile, I had a man with me. I never knew who he was. He couldn't tell me his name because when they first threw him into my cell his jaw was already so badly broken he couldn't speak. And it never healed. They made sure they beat him often enough so it wouldn't. *(A pause)* One night they brought him back, and I listened to him die. It took hours. *(A pause)* In the morning, when they brought that shit they feed us, I ate his too. When they came for him again, I dared them to take me instead. They were happy to oblige. Anyway, I kept them from finding out for a few days. I even dragged his body around the cell so when they looked in they'd think he was moving. *(A pause)* But then he started to smell, and... *(He shrugs)* They thought I'd gone crazy when I refused to give him up. They stood in the door with ther guns on me, cursing and shouting their lungs out...faces all red. I pulled him with me back against the wall, and I waited for them to shoot. *(A pause)* And nothing happened. *(Laughs)* I started to laugh at them standing there, watching me holding this dead man in my arms. The thing was... they were waiting, waiting for *me*, waiting to see what *I* would do. I still had choices, Oliver. *(A pause)* I could come to my senses, be a good Kaffir, and say "Ja, baas," and give him up. Or I could hold onto him until they came in and beat me. Or...I could walk

131

straight into their guns. *I* could make them be the monsters they were threatening to be. *(A pause)* Whatever happened would be because of the choice *I* made. Whatever they did would be in reaction to me. They were as bound by me as I by them because we were men in confrontation. *(A pause)* I was still a human being, and that was something all their laws and prisons and guns and power could not take away. Could never take away. *(A pause)* And I knew this was something our people needed to see. Something that would help them live, whether they got this... *freedom* they wanted or not.

I want her to keep the baby

CARELESS LOVE
by John Olive
Chicago - Present - Jack (early 30's)

Jack's young lover is pregnant and has decided to give the child up for adoption. When the reality of this situation finally sinks in, Jack explodes with anger and frustration.

JACK: So how's it work? You sign on the dotted line and they yank him out from between your legs, then carry him screaming through the double doors? Hand him to some stranger from the suburbs? "Bye. Have a nice one. Vote Democratic and thanks for the memories," just like that? Easy. *Degrade*

[MARTHA: Easy. You think it's gonna be easy? It'll be the hardest thing I'll ever have to do.]

[JACK: Then why are you doing it!]

[MARTHA: Because this is not a world that's very kind to twenty-year-old dancers with a baby, and no money, and no place to live. I'm not ready to be a mother, Jack if you thought about it, you'd see that.]

JACK: She's the only real thing I've ever done!

[MARTHA: She's not a thing! *(short pause)* She's not a thing.]

JACK: *(Pause. Sits on the sofa.)* Well. I guess it's the logical thing. Who are we, anyway? Actors, shit. It's all we can do to feed ourselves, much less some kid. Coupla crazy, kooky kids like us. Actors! *(quick beat)* Hey, there ya go. I bet they'll pay a real premium for our kid. A couple young, intelligent artists like us. Pretty. Healthy. White. That's important, isn't it? White people like us, most white people abort their mistakes, right? A pair of totally functional, top of the line adults like us, they'll pay top dollar. Whatever you do, for Christ sake, don't tell 'em I'm Irish Catholic, they'll knock twenty-five percent right off the top! *(stands)* You thief! Fucking sperm thief! The money and the time you've stolen from me, I've wasted nine months on you, you shit, you crazy little shit! And now you're gonna take it away from me, god damn it, and what'm I gonna do? My work is shit, Los Angeles

133

is shit, I'm nothing but shit! Marty! Marty! *(beat)* Please don't walk away from me. Everything I want's there in your belly. I don't have anything else. If you take it away, I'll die. I'll die. *(pauses)* I'll die. *(laughs)* Hey, look at me. Giving the performance of a lifetime. Too bad the Jeff Committee isn't here. I'm gonna be a star. A dream come true. I don't think I'll ever sleep again. *(beat)* I'm gonna die. *(JACK looks at MARTHA, then looks away.)* You better go to Sylvia's. Go on. I'll be okay. Go on. Go on!

EXECUTION OF JUSTICE
by Emily Mann
San Francisco - 1978-Present - Cop (40-50)

When Harvey Milk and George Moscone are gunned down by
Dan White, San Francisco is thrown into a period of violent
chaos. A conservative voice is heard here in the guise of a
policeman who wishes that things could be like they were in the
old days.

COP *(Quiet)*: Yeah, I'm wearing a "Free Dan White" T-shirt.
You haven't seen what I've seen—
my nose shoved into what I think stinks.
Against everything I believe in.
There was a time in San Francisco when you knew a guy
by his parish.
*(SISTER BOOM BOOM enters. Nun drag; white face, heavily made
up; spike heels.)*
Sometimes I sit in church and I think of those disgusting drag queens
dressed up as nuns and I'm a cop,
and I'm thinkin',
there's gotta be a law, you know,
because they're makin' me think things I don't want to think
and I gotta keep my mouth shut.
(BOOM BOOM puts out cigarette.)
Take a guy out of his sling—fist-fucked to death—
they say it's mutual consent, it ain't murder,
and I pull this disgusting mess down, take him to the morgue,
I mean, my wife asks me, "Hey, how was your day?"
I can't even tell her.
I wash my hands before I can even look at my kids.
*(The COP and BOOM BOOM are very aware of each other but
never make eye contact.)*
[BOOM BOOM: God bless you one. God bless you all.]
COP: See, Danny knew—he believes in the rights of minorities. Ya
know, he just felt—we are a minority, too.
[BOOM BOOM: I would like to open with a reading from the Book
of Dan. *(Opens book.)*]

EXECUTION OF JUSTICE

COP: We been workin' this job three generations—my father was
a cop—and then they put—Moscone, Jesus, Moscone put this
N-Negro-loving, faggot-loving Chief telling us what to do—
he doesn't even come from the neighborhood,
he doesn't even come from this city!
He's tellin' us what to do in a force that knows what to do.
He makes us paint our cop cars faggot blue—
he called it "lavender gloves" for the queers,
handle 'em, treat 'em with "lavender gloves," he called it.
He's cutting' off our balls.
The city is stinkin' with degenerates—
I mean, I'm worried about my kids, I worry about my wife,
I worry about me and how I'm feelin' mad all the time.
You gotta understand that I'm not alone—
It's real confusion.
[BOOM BOOM: "As he came to his day of reckoning, he feared
not for he went unto the lawyers and the doctors and the jurors, and
they said, 'Take heart, for in this you will receive not life but three
to seven with time off for good behavior.'" *(Closes book
reverently)*]
COP: Ya gotta understand—
Take a walk with me sometime.
See what I see every day...
[BOOM BOOM: Now we are all faced with this cycle.]
COP: Like I'm supposed to smile when I see two bald-headed,
shaved-head men with those tight pants and muscles,
chains everywhere, french-kissin' on the street,
putting their hands all over each other's asses,
I'm supposed to smile,
walk by, act as if this is *right??!!*
[BOOM BOOM: As gay people and as people of color and as
women we all know the cycle of brutality which pervades our
culture.]
COP: I got nothin' against people doin' what they want, if I don't
see it.

GONE THE BURNING SUN
by Ken Mitchell
Michigan - 1930 - Dr. Norman Bethune (30-40)

Bethune was a Canadian physican whose passionate political beliefs brought him to field hospitals in the Spanish Civil War and the Chinese Resistance during the Japanese invasion of 1930. Here, the outspoken young doctor visits a friend in Michigan and laspes into a provocatively metaphysical monologue.

BETHUNE: Barney? You home? Barnwell, you old zombie! Might've known you'd emerge from this elegant woodwork somewhere! No, no special reason. Drove all the way to Michigan just to bend a friend's ear. Yeah. I depend on you to laugh at my jokes, Barney—hell, you're the only one who even listens to me. Got any whiskey?

(removes the scarf, takes a glass)

Cheers. Oh—you heard. Yes, Frannie and I married again. November. Wonderful ceremony. Only two years after the divorce. Romantic, eh? Frances *loved* it—far more sentimental than I. Hmm? Oh—no, it's bust again, I'm sad to say. No, the same old story. Can't reconcile our irreconcilable natures. We get along beauti-fully—as long as we're not together. Oh, she's taking it all "splendidly." Now she's off the kirk again—to marry our best man. Coleman—an old pal of mine, I think you met in Montreal. I'm sure they'll be very happy. No, no—we're all great friends.

Barney, don't try to understand me. You never did before—and you always understood perfectly.

Well—yes. Fit as a fiddle, I suppose. Thirty miles on skis, every weekend. I know the Laurentians better than my own bronchial tubes. Regular workouts in the gym. I do my own artificial pneumothorax now—can't trust my homicidal colleagues. I've been fine-tuning the machine. Want to see?

(He removes a machine from his suitcase and places it on the table.)

GONE THE BURNING SUN

(He removes his jacket and shirt.)

Well—according to the gout-gang at the Royal Vic, this is dangerous lunacy. Self-treatment. Aaah, I don't fit in there, Barney. I think my career in lung surgery may be coming to an end. You have a clean needle in your case there, Dr. Barnwell? Thanks.

(inserts a large hypodermic needle into a tube)

Novocain? Naah—don't believe in that stuff.

(plunges the needle into his chest)

There—between the sixth—and seventh ribs. Now pump the air— into the chest—around the lung.

(coughs painfully, jerks the needle out, grins)

There. Collapsed. "One-lung Bethune" they call me in the *brasseries* of the Old Town.

(puts the machine away, dresses again)

Afraid? Of death? *Me?* Barney, I intend to die of an overdose of sex at the age of ninety. *(laughs, coughs)* Of course, I'm serious! When I joke—I'm serious! You know that. All right, maybe I'm a bit—lost. I thought I was onto something when I went to Montreal! Surgery for surgery's sake. Cut and be damned. But Christ, Barney— the odds! We need more effective ways of fighting T.B. Now—the *cause* of disease—if we could just eliminate that, eh? You know, there are two kinds of T.B. The rich man's T.B.—and the poor man's. The rich man recovers. The poor man dies. And that's it! We need the Depression before it suddenly becomes obvious. So why are we scrambling for a cure in the medical lab? Now we have social tools—and we've got to cut out the cause. There *has* to be a way—right? And I have this sense— just an intuition—ever since I left the San—that Bethune is part of it. Oh, I dunno—maybe there's some sort of "cosmic adventure" directing my life. Sure it worries me—and it's really hard on my friends, I know—Frances, you. Afraid of destroying them in my rush to destroy myself. Oh yes—that's what people are saying! "Look out for Bethune. A bomb—looking for a place to explode." No, don't deny it! I know things about myself that people should never know.

GONE THE BURNING SUN

(pours another drink, hesitating)

Remember the time I disappeared from the Sanitorium for two days? Frances was back then, after the operation—I got a letter from her in New York—she'd met up with some rich playboy—he was treating her badly. I dunno, looking back—maybe she made all that up. But I went nuts. I always said I was never jealous, but—there I was on the train, going after this chump—planning how to—kill him. *(laughs)* Twenty bucks in my pocket. Spitting slugs of fuchsia-coloured snot all over the aisle. Got to town at seven in the morning, up to Harlem, bought a gun. Registered in some hotel. God, I musta looked like a vampire. I rang him up, anyway—gave him a phoney name, some "long lost friend from Princeton." *Insisted* he come down to the hotel for a drink. Sat down to wait.

(sits, draws an imaginary gun)

"Come in! No. No mistake. I'm Norman Bethune. Beth. Une. Thaaaaat's right—Frannie's husband. I'm here exterminating pests." *(stands)* "So—anything to say? *Nothing?* You did screw her, didn't you? Well, don't just stand there, trembling. Defend yourself!" *(advances, hesitates)* "You deserve it? Well, I'll be goddamned— if—that isn't—the mingiest goddamn limp-wristed excuse—"

(BETHUNE suddenly strikes him with the "gun.")

"So, does that stiffen the old backbone? No?"

(BETHUNE hits him several times, going crazy. He stops, coughing violently. He hurls the "gun" away.)

"Aaaa! Get out!"

(calms down)

"Come on—get up on your feet. And quit that awful *bawling!* I *hate* cry-babies! Here—sit down. Ah, that's a nasty cut. There's a towel"

(extends his scarf)

"God, what a mess. Well, you can't go down to the lobby looking like this—"

(turns back to BARNWELL, lights a cigarette)

GONE THE BURNING SUN

Anyway, we drank a bottle of Jack Daniels, got into dirty limericks—sent him home in a taxi. Came back on the train that night. So—you see what I mean. Crazy, eh? And I cannot inflict this sort of thing on my friends. My few friends.

Oh, but I thought Montreal was the answer! The gay bachelor's life. Beautiful women—dozens of them. Plenty of hard work. I paint, I teach—even started writing poetry! A good life but—not enough. Still not enough.

I think sometimes I'm really an *artist*, trapped in a doctor's body. There I am standing in front of this canvas of living flesh, scalpel and palette in hand. Now you see why my colleagues think I'm dangerous. I am, too. Oh, you know what I mean. An artist has to *let go*—abandon himself to action. He comes up into the light like some "creature of the monstrous deep"—all jagged and destructive— breaking the smooth surface of mediocrity. And in the banal glare of day, he *enjoys* the purification of violence.

Of course, it's disturbing! The artist's *function* is to disturb! His duty is to rouse the sleeping. To shake the pillars of the world! He must remind humans of their dark ancestry, and still direct them toward a new birth.

I'm no reformer, Barney. I'm a revolutionary! In a world already terrified of change, I preach *revolution!* The principle of life! I am a disturber of the excrement—an agitator—impatient—frightening! I am the creative spirit, liberating the soul of men!

(collapses on the table, drunk)

Where can a guy take a leak, Barney?

(staggers toward the exit)

HURLYBURLY
by David Rabe
Hollywood - Present - Eddie (30's)

Early morning finds Eddie, Phil and Mickey struggling to begin another day in L.A. Phil has just left his wife, Eddie is suffering from a terrible coke hangover and Mickey just wishes there was something to eat in the house. Eddie, a coke-addicted casting director thoroughly desensitized by life, needs to do a line of coke just to wake up and here comes to life after a snort.

EDDIE: *(Clearly snubbing MICKEY, EDDIE turns to PHIL, who is spooning coke from the vial.)* I gotta wake up. *(as PHIL puts the coke to one of EDDIE's nostrils)* I got a lot of work today. *(PHIL puts coke to Eddie's other nostril and EDDIE snorts, then grabs PHIL's face between his hands.)* The shit that went down here last night was conspiratorial. *(EDDIE leaps to his feet, putting on his glasses and grabbing the newspaper from the end table. Jolted with the coke, he is a whirlwind of information.)* First of all the eleven o'clock news has just devastated me with this shitload of horror in which it sounds like not only are we headed for nuclear devastation if not by the Russians then by some goddamn primitive bunch of middle-eastern motherfuckers— *(Pacing behind the couch, he roots through the paper, while PHIL watches and MICKEY, abandoned in the kitchen nook, eats the snowball.)* —and I don't mean that racially but just culturally, because they are so far back in the forest in some part of their goddamn mental sophistication, they are likely to drop the bomb just to see the light and hear the big noise. I mean, I am talking not innate ability, but sophistication here. They have got to get off the camels and wake up! *(Handing the newspapers to PHIL, EDDIE starts up the stairs.)* So on top of this, there's this accidental electrical fire in which an entire family is incinerated, the father trying to save everybody by hurling them out the window, but he's on the sixth floor, so they're like eggs on the sidewalk. So much for heroics. So then my wife calls! You wanna have some absurdity?

HURLYBURLY
by David Rabe
Hollywood - Present - Phil (30's)

Phil is a struggling LA actor who has recently left his wife. His contempt for women becomes evident when he verbally attacks Donna, a sixteen year-old waif who trades sex for a place to sleep, for distracting him from watching a football game on TV.

PHIL: What makes you tick? I come here to see Eddie, you gotta be here. I wanna watch the football game and talk over some very important issues which pertain to my life, you gotta be here. What the fuck makes you tick?

[DONNA: What's he talkin' about?]

[EDDIE: I don't know.]

[PHIL: What I'm talkin' about is—]

[EDDIE: *(Stepping in front of him as he moves toward DONNA.)* Listen, Phil, if Darlene comes by, you just introduce Donna as your ditz, okay? He starts up the stairs for his room.]

[DONNA: Who's Darlene, Phil?]

PHIL: *(His hands up in surrender, he retreats into the kitchen.)* I'm beggin' you. I'm beggin' you. I don't wanna see you, okay? I don't wanna see you.

[DONNA: Okay.]

PHIL: *(grabbing his beer and bowl of popcorn)* I mean, I come in here and you gotta be here; I'm thinkin' about football, and you gotta be here with your tits and your ass and this tight shrunken clothes and these shriveled jeans, so that's all I'm thinking about from the minute I see you is tits and ass. Football doesn't have a chance against it. It's like this invasion of tits and ass overwhelming my own measly individuality so I don't have a prayer to have my own thoughts about my own things except you and tits and ass and sucking and fucking and that's all I can think about. My privacy has been demolished. *(Sitting down next to her on the couch. As he talks, she nibbles his popcorn.)* You think a person wants to have that kind of thing happen to their heads—they are trying to give their own problems serious thought, the next thing they know there's nothing in their brains as far as they can see but your tits and ass? You think a person likes that?

142

THE INCREDIBLY FAMOUS WILLY RIVERS
by Stephen Metcalfe
Here and Now - Willy (30's)

Willy Rivers is a rock star who is struggling to make a comeback after an attempt has been made on his life. Willy was shot during the attack and is no longer able to play the guitar as he used to. Here, he tries to explain the magic of making music to a man in a three piece suit.

WILLY: I started off playing to records. Man, I'd turn the stereo up to a thousand and I'd dance with that first guitar of mine like it was my baby. Mom had a headache from the mid-sixties on. Why do you play the stereo so loud, Willy!? You're gonna ruin your eardrums! She never understood that loud is the only way rock and roll sounds good. She was also convinced I woulda turned out normal if the Beatles hadn't been on Ed Sullivan. She didn't think I did teenage things. Go out with a girl, Willy! Get her pregnant. Go total a car! Go protest something like all your other friends! Go protest traffic lights, Doberman pinschers. Go protest bell-bottom pants! My mom prayed for a moment's peace. Now my dad, my dad sorta knew how much it all meant to me. Course he didn't have to listen to it all day long. But he'd come home and let Mom blow off steam for awhile and then he'd come down to the basement and he'd look at the posters I'd taped to the walls, black-light crazy shit, and he'd turn to me and he'd say, go for it, Willy. For your mom's sake, go for it quietly but go for it. My dad...he was a fan. *(HE strikes a chord. It sounds rough and tinny)* That was an A chord, man. The perfect A chord. I learned a chord a day. Perfect chords. I practiced till my fingers bled. All that practice... And man? I can't play worth a shit anymore. *(Flexing his hand, putting down the guitar)* Nerve damage.
[SUIT: You're a headliner now, Willy, you don't have to play. Others will play for you. All you have to do is stand there and look good.]
[WILLY: Hey...maybe I should mouth the words too?]

143

THE INCREDIBLY FAMOUS WILLY RIVERS

[SUIT: We can arrange that if you like.]
WILLY: [You're never gonna understand.] When you play the sound right, it's like stepping into another plane of existence, man. Your body is pistons, tubes, valves. You're aware of rods flowing into cylinders, of liquid seeping from chamber into chamber, of billows as they fill and empty, of life, man! You're aware of the tiny delicate bones in the inner room of your ear, of filaments dancing to the pulse of a beat. You hear with your heart when you play, man. The music speaks words, man. You are, man. Man!

THE UNDOING
by William Mastrosimone
Poultry shop - Present - Berk (30-40)

Berk is hired by Lorraine to kill chickens in her poultry shop. Lorraine is an alcoholic desperate for salvation and Berk becomes determined to help her to quit drinking. Lorraine's husband was killed by a drunk driver: Berk. In a highly emotional confrontation, Berk finally admits to being the driver of the car that killed her husband.

BERK: I twisted in my hospital bed till the I.V. tubes pulled out. Nurses saved me every time. I lay there seven months...jaw wired...couldn't talk...or see...or move...alone with myself and the sound of the man in that wreck... I read his obituary... "Survived by his wife Lorraine Tempesta and their daughter."... They had to strap me down. I kept pulling the tubes out to stop that voice of the man in the wreck screaming... They kept saving me. They told me I was lucky. Another quarter inch and I'd be an asparagus. I bumped wheelchairs with the terminal ill, double amputees who only had a cup of soup and maybe a chair in the sun to hope for. I was only a quarter inch from being one of the slobbering morons who talked twenty-four hours to the air, to memories, and I knew I had to save myself from that... I knew I had to forgive myself to stop the sound of that voice of the man in the wreck...or dive out my window...somebody already thought of that...it was barred...but that wasn't enough to stop the voice... "Survived by his wife Lorraine Tempesta and their daughter"... I called from my hospital room... I hung up when I heard your voice say, "Leo's"... I wanted to say something to you... But what could I say? I thought I should get the chair...but the judge fined me five hundred dollars...took away my license for a year...for murder—murder! They didn't punish me, so I punished myself... So I came here. I saw you in your bloody apron, gizzard in your hair, liver stains on your fingers, bloodshot eyes... You thought I came for a job... The scream of the man in the car wreck stopped... Stopped... That's what the sign said... STOP... I wanted to give back something... I gave you my life... I didn't have anything else to give.

BABY WITH THE BATHWATER
by Christopher Durang
Here and Now - Daisy (17)

Daisy is a young man who has been raised as a girl by his parents. Here, he begins to tell his tale to an unseen voice which somewhat resembles that of a psychoanalyst. As he speaks, Daisy begins to reveal details from his horrific childhood. Truly chilling, however, is his matter of fact descriptions of such a criminally distorted situation.

DAISY: [Well, probably. It all got straightened out eventually.] When I was eleven, I came across this medical book that had pictures in it, and I realized that I looked more like a boy than a girl, but my mother had always wanted a girl or a best-seller, and I didn't want to disappoint her. But then some days, I don't know what gets into me, I would just feel like striking out at them. So I'd wait till she was having one of her crying fits, and I took the book to her—I was twelve now—and I said, Have you ever seen this book? Are you totally insane? Why have you named me Daisy? Everyone else has always said I was a boy, what's the *matter* with you? And she kept crying and she said something about Judith Krantz and then she said, I want to die; and then she said, *perhaps* you're a boy, but we don't want to jump to any hasty conclusions, so why don't we just wait, and we'd see if I menstruated or not. And I asked her what that word meant, and she slapped me and washed my mouth out with soap. Then she apologized and hugged me, and said she was a bad mother. Then she washed *her* mouth out with soap. Then she tied me to the kitchen table and turned on all the gas jets and said it would be just a little while longer for the both of us. Then my father came home and he turned off the gas jets and untied me. Then when he asked if dinner was ready, she lay on the kitchen floor and wouldn't move, and he said, I guess not, and then he sort of crouched next to the refrigerator and tried to read a book, but I don't think he was really reading, because he never turned any of the pages. And then eventually, since nothing else seemed to be happening, I just went to bed.

146

THE DOG
by David Mamet
Here and Now - Man (20-50)

Here, a regular kind of guy describes his relationship with his dog.

MAN: Talk about a dog! Talk about a precious animal! A little fluffball. A furry little nothing. But ballsy as a paratrooper.

He's tough, but I'm *tougher*. Benjy may be tough but I'm yet tougher.

Go after dogs twice his size. Three, four times his size. Go right up to 'em. Sniff 'em. Smell 'em up and down...

He growls, bares his teeth.

He scares 'em. He's little, but goddamn it if he's not a scrapper. And they know it. Damn right they do, too.

Sensitive?

He's more sensitive than most *people*. Makes most people look sick, he's so sensitive. In tune like a human.

He picks up on things, too.

I come home, he meets me at the door. Grinning, breathing fast, he's glad to see me.

I got to hang up my coat, and what do I find? The little pisser has shit on the floor! He's crossed me. My best friend has crossed me.

So I go over to him, he's grinning like a sonofabitch, and I say *sit*. And he sits down and cocks his head, wondering what's up.

I make a fist, and lean over and whack the shit outta him. He goes clear across the room and just lays there on his side.

So then I say *get up* and he gets up. And I say *sit* and he sits down again and I walk over to him.

So he's purebred, he's no dummy. And he figures maybe I'm going to knock him around again, and he's a little scared.

But he hangs right in there.

I say *stay*. And it's like he's glued to the floor. He'd sit there for a year if I didn't tell him different.

THE DOG

So I go over and get a chair and bring it back and put it right in front of him. I sit down, lean back, and cross my legs.

I look at him. He looks at me.

After a minute or so, I lean forward and say, very reasonable and soft, I say "Don't shit on the floor. Now, get outta here."

And I never have to say a word on the subject again.

K2
by Patrick Meyers
A mountain ledge - September 4, 1977 - Taylor (30-40)

Survival is the name of the game for two men stranded on a narrow ledge located on a 600 foot ice wall at 27,000 feet on K2, the world's second highest mountain. Harold's broken leg makes it impossible for him to assist Taylor in any plan to escape. When an argument regarding the best way for Taylor to got for help ensues, the voltile Taylor explodes at his friend, revealing years of pent-up frustration and resentment.

TAYLOR: Listen, Harold, you don't know what's goin' on down there all around you every day, every night—while you sleep, make love with Cindy, eat Chinese food, play with atoms at Lawrence Radiation Center. All around you all the time, you don't know buddy. Sure you read about some of it in the papers, selected atrocities for your viewing pleasure, Stew, Earl, all a ya, sittin' around bitchin' about crime in the neighborhood and social injustice all the same breath. Christ, if you guys had any idea of what's really goin' on out there under your fuckin' noses, you'd be so damn scared you'd shit and die...there's a war goin' on down there—and the barbarians are winning! They're kickin' our civilized asses all over the streets...you know that out of every ten faces I prosecute—one is white, two are brown, and the other seven are black? What does that tell you Harold?
[HAROLD: What do you think it tells me?]
[TAYLOR: I'm asking.]
[HAROLD: It's not a real tough one to read Taylor...we're a racist society.]
TAYLOR: "A racist society"... That's just the self-consciously hip answer I would expect from a white middle class liberal. I'm not talking about moral culpability you frigging clown, I'm talking about what is. I'm talking about what the fuck is going on. You think makin' the free lunch a little bigger some kind of real swell humanitarian act don't you? That's the way to solve the problem

149

right? Hmmm? *(Harold does not respond.)* Let me tell you what your god damn bigger and better free lunch has produced. It's produced a black male, average age thirteen to twenty-five, average weight one hundred and thirty to two hundred and twenty pounds, who has the reflexes of a rattler, the strength of a rhino, and the compassion of a pit bull. He can rip off you and your grandma before you can count to one and he'll take it all—your money, your clothes, your assholes—both of 'em—and he'll get her false teeth! That's what you get when you take away somebody's dignity and try to make it up to 'em by givin' 'em a free bag of goceries and a place to sleep...and I put 'em away every day. I make sure they get their three squares and a place to flop behind fifty foot walls with some gun towers up top. That's what you pay me to do Harold, and I do it extremely well. I do it to clean up after all you pollyanna jerks... I do it for you and Cindy, Harold. I do it to "protect and serve" what little of our society is left.

COUP/CLUCKS
by Jane Martin
Brine, Alabama - Present - Don (30's)

As all of Brine, Alabama prepares for the annual Tara Parade and Ball, Don, the local hairdresser, helps Miz Zifty to make the transformation from dowdy old Southern Belle to Scarlett O'Hara lookalike. Miz Zifty has played the part of Scarlett in the parade for years, and only Don can help her to capture the essence of the role. Here, he chatters as he works.

DON: *(Working on MIZ ZIFTY's hair)* Why did I come back to Brine, Alabama? Leave the bright lights of New York City? Cowardice, I suppose. I swear, wherever I go I feel like a fly in a frogpond. Victim-in-residence. They ever made a movie about me they'd call it "Born to Shake." Makes me just furious I can't change my nature. Know who I'm comin' back as in my next life? John Wayne. *(Handing her a mirror)* Here, peek.
[MIZ ZIFTY: *(Doubtfully)* Well...]
DON: Darlin', you're the personification, that's what you are.
[MIZ ZIFTY: You'd think the very least the Good Lord could have done would have been to make old age pretty.]
DON: [Oh, poo.] If Ashley Wilkes doesn't nibble you like a praline, the man's a stone. So, anyway, I'd quit my hair stylin' job 'cause I was petrified to take the subway, and there I was, catatonic in Times Square, appalled by the sheer unendurable ugliness, transfixed by the lack, the absence of any beauty, anything soothing to the soul, when suddenly I was struck from behind...hard enough to see stars. I turn, and there is a wild man, a Martian savage dressed entirely in debris. Had on plastic Clorox bottles for shoes, white garbage bags wrapped for leggins, cardboard mailing tubes on his arms, face caked with filth, plus he had on, so help me Hannah, an actual medieval breastplate. Like out of a museum, darlin'. And this staff he struck me with is covered with "Nixon's the One" buttons. Well his wild blue eyes lock with mine, he grabs my Pierre Cardin tie, shakes me like a rag doll and shrieks in my face, "Why

don't you weirdos get the hell out of New York City!"
[MIZ ZIFTY: That doesn't surprise you I hope. That's normal
Yankee behavior.]
*(BEULAH, MIZ ZIFTY's sixty-year-old black maid, enters, carrying
a tray which holds several bowls of finger-foods. She places them
about the room.)*
DON: Well, I fled, darlin', fled home to Brine. Our rednecks may
be mean, dumb, and violent, but at least they are not dressed in
medieval breastplates. You seen 'em on the square this mornin'?
Waiting t'laugh y'all to shame?

COUP/CLUCKS
by Jane Martin
Brine, Alabama - Present - Ryman (30-40)

Ryman is a Klan member in a small town in Brine, Alabama.
Ryman has some very strange ideas about black people and time,
as he here describes while assembling a bomb.

RYMAN: *(Still tinkering with screwdriver and pliers inside the tool
box, which contains a bomb)* White man's down to the last tick of
the clock. Last mother tick. All a man's got is time. You don't
have time, you don't have nothin' but rigor mortis. You see this
here decade-calendar, stop-sequence, microselective, astro-
chronometer, digital-watch? White man designed this. Time's only
in the white man's mind. Ain't no colored ever designed a good
watch. Why you think they call it "colored people's time"? 'Cause
it's late. Why you think there ain't no colored people in
Switzerland? 'Cause that's where they make the watches. They
lettin' us live fast while they live slow so they can be here when
we're gone, brothers! They screwin' aroun' with our life span.
Stealin' the white man's time. Got them a warehouse full of our
minutes. An' our only hope...the only hope is the microprocessor,
so we'll know exactly where we are down to the millisecond, an'
they know it. Them spades made themselves up like Japanese an'
snuck into I.B.M. t'steal that program, an' if the security guard
hadn't noticed they was wearin' bright maroon platform shoes, that
woulda' been all she wrote, brother! They ain't gonna get our time!
Ain't gonna steal our life! I got a surprise for the colored, brothers.
You see if I don't.

CLOUD NINE
by Caryl Churchill
London - 1980 - Gerry (20-30)

Gerry tells his lover, Edward, that he needs to go to the pub to
clear his head after a minor spat. On his way, he describes a
sexual encounter that he recently experienced on a train.

GERRY: [I didn't ask you to come.] *(to audience)* You have to
get away sometimes or you lose sight of yourself. The train from
Victoria to Clapham is one of the old type. Separate compartments,
no connecting corridor, so once the train starts no one can get in or
out until the next station. As soon as I got on the platform I saw
who I wanted. Slim hips, tense shoulders, trying not to look at
anyone. I put my hand on my packet just long enough so he
couldn't miss it. The train came in. You don't want to get in too
fast or some straight dumbo might get in with you. I stay by the
window. I couldn't see where the fuck he'd got to. Then just as the
whistle went he got in. Great. It's a six-minute journey so you
can't start anything you can't finish. I stared at him and he unzipped
his flies. Then he stopped. So I stood up and took my cock out.
He took me in his mouth and shut his eyes tight. He was sort of
mumbling it about as if he wasn't sure what to do, so I said, "A bit
tighter son" and he said "Sorry" and then got on with it. He was
jerking off with his left hand, and I could see he's got a fair-sized
one. I wished he'd keep still so I could see his watch. I was getting
really turned on. What if we pull into Clapham Junction now. Of
course by the time we sat down again the train was just slowing up.
I felt wonderful. Then he started talking. It's better if nothing is
said. Once you find he's a librarian in Walthamstow with a special
interest in science fiction and lives with his aunt, then forget it. He
said I hope you don't think I do this all the time. I said I hope you
will from now on. He said he would if I was on the train, but why
don't we go out for a meal? I opened the door before the train
stopped. I told him I live with somebody, I don't want to know. He
was jogging sideways to keep up. He said "what's your phone

154

number, you're my ideal physical type, what sign of the zodiac are you? Where do you live? Where are you going now? It's not fair."
I saw him at Victoria a couple of months later and I went straight down to the end of the platform and I picked up somebody really great who never said a word. Just smiled.

ARISTOCRATS
by Brian Friel
Ireland - Summer, 1970's - Eamon (30's)

The O'Donnell family has gathered at their ancestral home in Ballybeg for a wedding. Joining them is an American academic who is writing a thesis on the Catholic aristocracy in Ireland. Eamon, a local who married into the O'Donnell clan here reveals his resentment of the decaying class structure in Ireland.

EAMON: My grandmother. You'd find her interesting. Worked all her life as a maid here in the Hall.

[TOM: In the Hall? Here?]

EAMON: Didn't you know that? Oh, yes, yes. Something like fifty-seven years continuous service with the District Justice and his wife, Lord have mercy on her; and away back to the earlier generation, with his father, the High Court judge and his family. Oh, you should meet her before you leave—a fund of stories and information.

[TOM: She sounds—]

EAMON: Carriages, balls, receptions, weddings, christenings, feasts, deaths, trips to Rome, musical evenings, tennis—that's the mythology I was nurtured on all my life, day after day, year after year—the life of the 'quality'—that's how she pronounces it, with a flat 'a'. A strange and marvellous education for a wee country boy, wasn't it? No, not an education—a permanent pigmentation. I'll tell you something, Professor: I know more about this place, infinitely more, here and here, (head and heart) than they know. Sure? *(drink)* You'll enjoy this. *(Now to ALICE up in the gazebo)* Telling the professor about the night I told granny you and I were getting married. *(To TOM)* Not a notion in the world we were going out, of course. My God, Miss Alice and her grandson! Anyhow, 'Granny', I said this night, 'Alice and I are going to get married'. 'Alice? Who's Alice? Alice Devenny? Alice Byrne? Not Alice Smith!' 'Alice O'Donnell'. 'What Alice O'Donnell's that?' 'Alice O'Donnell of the Hall'. A long silence. Then: 'May God and his holy mother forgive you, you dirty-mouthed upstart!' *(Laughs)*. Wasn't that an interesting response? As we say about here: Now you're an educated man, Professor—what do make of that response?

156

COLUMBUS AVENUE
by David Mamet
Columbus Avenue - Present - Man (50-60)

An older merchant here gets a harsh dose of reality when he is
evicted from his place of business.

MAN: I felt the cold steel of a gun against my head three times.

Twenty-six years we have been here. A tailor fourteen years
before that here. Fifty-one years.

And he's an Orthodox Jew, and his father said (when he was
managing: when first we settled on a price; and, you know, we
negotiated...but when we were done he told me): "I will never
throw you out."

The boy, he said, "Before I do a thing we'll talk." Today I get
his letter in the mail. And I go there. I say, "You said that we
were going to talk." He said, "I thought instead of talking I'd send
you a letter."

So what am I going to do? Where am I going to go?

My customers are going to follow me? Can I ask them to walk
for twenty blocks?

If even he gave me a *ten*-year lease, at least then I could sell the
business.

So I said *double* the rent. *Triple* the rent, I told him.

He has got a *guy* is going to pay two thousand a month, he says.
And he's going to put in fifty-thousand dollars restoration.

I told him, "How is he going to make the *rent*?"

He said, "He'll break his back. He'll break his back the first
year," (he didn't say "back") "and, after that, he *fails*, I've got his
fifty thousand he put in my building, and I rent the place again."

It's like the whole street: Things you don't want at what you
can't afford, and nothing that you need.

No services.

Where am I going to go?

If I was twenty, if I was even ten years *younger*...

Where am I going to go? I got to move the *press*, I got to move the *racks*; by the time I put *in* I put in all my savings to the *business* to go somewhere else and I have nothing. And I have to start again. Twenty-six years.

I told him, "I hate to remind you what your father said."
He shrugged.

My *wife* went. I was getting sick. He said he'd give us an extension for six months.

It's the same all the neighborhood.

Let the depression come, and see who pays the rent.

Twenty-six years I've been here, and there are no more services on this street anymore.

What will people do I don't know what he thinks.

I don't know.

I don't know what I can say.

THE DRESSER
by Ronald Harwood
English Theater - 1942 - Sir (60's)

This aging and ailing Shakesperian actor takes a moment during an intermission of "King Lear" to reflect upon his performance in the role that has eluded him for so long. He is at the end of his career and his life, much like the tragic king which he portrays.

SIR: I'm not well, I have half of Lear's lifetime yet to live, I have to lift you in my arms, I have howl, howl, howl yet to speak.
[HER LAYDYSHIP: Sir. Her Ladyship. We're a laughing-stock. You'd never get a knighthood because the King doesn't possess a double-edged sword. The only honour you'll ever get is when you go on stage and we all bow.]
(Silence)
SIR: I thought tonight I caught sight of him. Or saw myself as he sees me. Speaking 'Reason not the need,' I was suddenly detached from myself. My thoughts flew. And I was observing from a great height. Go on, you bastard, I seemed to be saying or hearing. Go on, you've more to give, don't hold back more, more, more. And I was watching Lear. Each word he spoke was fresh invented. I had no knowledge of what came next, what fate awaited him. The agony was in the moment of acting created. I saw an old man and the old man was me. And I knew there was more to come. But what? Bliss, partial recovery, more pain and death. All this I knew I had yet to see. Outside myself, do you understand? Outside myself. *(HE holds out his hand. SHE does not take it)* Don't leave me. I'll rest easy if you stay. Don't ask of me the impossible. Otherwise, I know, without you, in darkness, I'll see a locked door, a sign turned in the window, closed, gone away, and a drawn blind.

159

161

162

163

169

Smith and Kraus *Books For Actors*

THE MONOLOGUE SERIES
The Best Men's / Women's Stage Monologues of 1994
The Best Men's / Women's Stage Monologues of 1993
The Best Men's / Women's Stage Monologues of 1992
The Best Men's / Women's Stage Monologues of 1991
The Best Men's / Women's Stage Monologues of 1990
One Hundred Men's / Women's Stage Monologues from the 1980's
2 Minutes and Under: Character Monologues for Actors
Street Talk: Character Monologues for Actors
Uptown: Character Monologues for Actors
Ice Babies in Oz: Character Monologues for Actors
Monologues from Contemporary Literature: Volume I
Monologues from Classic Plays
100 Great Monologues from the Renaissance Theatre
100 Great Monologues from the Neo-Classical Theatre
100 Great Monologues from the 19th C. Romantic and Realistic Theatres
A Brave and Violent Theatre: 20th C. Irish Monologues, Scenes & Hist. Context
Kiss and Tell: Restoration Monologues, Scenes and Historical Context
The Great Monologues from the Humana Festival
The Great Monologues from the EST Marathon
The Great Monologues from the Women's Project
The Great Monologues from the Mark Taper Forum

YOUNG ACTOR SERIES
Great Scenes and Monologues for Children
Great Monologues for Young Actors
Great Scenes for Young Actors from the Stage
Multicultural Scenes for Young Actors
Multicultural Monologues for Young Actors

SCENE STUDY SERIES
Scenes From Classic Plays 468 B.C. to 1960 A.D.
The Best Stage Scenes of 1995
The Best Stage Scenes of 1994
The Best Stage Scenes of 1993
The Best Stage Scenes of 1992
The Best Stage Scenes for Men / Women from the 1980's

If you require pre-publication information about upcoming Smith and Kraus books, you may receive our semi-annual catalogue, free of charge, by sending your name and address to *Smith and Kraus Catalogue, P.O. Box 127, One Main Street, Lyme, NH 03768. Or call us at (800) 895-4331, fax (603) 795-4427.*